# CSF Rhinorrhea

T0136337

# CSF Rhinorrhea

## Management and Practice

Editor-in-Chief

## Jyotirmay S Hegde

Associate Editor

## Hemanth Vamanshankar

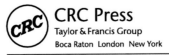

CRC Press
Taylor & Francis Group
Boca Raton London New York

CRC Press is an imprint of the
Taylor & Francis Group, an **informa** business

Illustrations in Chapters 2, 4, 5, 6 and 14 were conceptualized and created by the associate editor Dr Hemanth Vamanshankar.

First edition published 2021

by CRC Press
6000 Broken Sound Parkway NW, Suite 300, Boca Raton, FL 33487-2742

and by CRC Press
2 Park Square, Milton Park, Abingdon, Oxon, OX14 4RN

© 2021 Taylor & Francis Group, LLC
CRC Press is an imprint of Taylor & Francis Group, LLC

This book contains information obtained from authentic and highly regarded sources. While all reasonable efforts have been made to publish reliable data and information, neither the author[s] nor the publisher can accept any legal responsibility or liability for any errors or omissions that may be made. The publishers wish to make clear that any views or opinions expressed in this book by individual editors, authors or contributors are personal to them and do not necessarily reflect the views/opinions of the publishers. The information or guidance contained in this book is intended for use by medical, scientific or health-care professionals and is provided strictly as a supplement to the medical or other professional's own judgement, their knowledge of the patient's medical history, relevant manufacturer's instructions and the appropriate best practice guidelines. Because of the rapid advances in medical science, any information or advice on dosages, procedures or diagnoses should be independently verified. The reader is strongly urged to consult the relevant national drug formulary and the drug companies' and device or material manufacturers' printed instructions, and their websites, before administering or utilizing any of the drugs, devices or materials mentioned in this book. This book does not indicate whether a particular treatment is appropriate or suitable for a particular individual. Ultimately it is the sole responsibility of the medical professional to make his or her own professional judgements, so as to advise and treat patients appropriately. The authors and publishers have also attempted to trace the copyright holders of all material reproduced in this publication and apologize to copyright holders if permission to publish in this form has not been obtained. If any copyright material has not been acknowledged please write and let us know so we may rectify in any future reprint.

Except as permitted under U.S. Copyright Law, no part of this book may be reprinted, reproduced, transmitted, or utilized in any form by any electronic, mechanical, or other means, now known or hereafter invented, including photocopying, microfilming, and recording, or in any information storage or retrieval system, without written permission from the publishers.

For permission to photocopy or use material electronically from this work, access www.copyright.com or contact the Copyright Clearance Center, Inc. (CCC), 222 Rosewood Drive, Danvers, MA 01923, 978-750-8400. For works that are not available on CCC please contact mpkbookspermissions@tandf.co.uk

*Trademark notice*: Product or corporate names may be trademarks or registered trademarks and are used only for identification and explanation without intent to infringe.

*Library of Congress Cataloging-in-Publication Data*
Cataloging-in-Publication data are on file in the Library of Congress.

ISBN: 9780367029630 (hbk)
ISBN: 9780367029586 (pbk)
ISBN: 9780429019814 (ebk)

Typeset in Minion
by Deanta Global Publishing Services, Chennai, India

Visit the eResources: www.routledge.com/9780367029586.

To

My beloved grandmother – Paiamma

Jyotirmay S Hegde

My parents, brother, wife and all my teachers – for what I am today.

Hemanth Vamanshankar

# Contents

# Foreword

## DIFFICULT SUBJECT MADE RIDICULOUSLY SIMPLE

It is indeed a great pleasure and a proud moment for me to be writing the foreword for the book of one of the best postgraduate students we ever had in the Department of Otolaryngology – Head and Neck Surgery at Karnataka Institute of Medical Sciences, Hubli. I have known Jyotirmay for 15 years now and have seen him grow and attain great heights in his career. He is a disciplinarian and a silent achiever.

The surgical procedures of endoscopic anterior skull base surgery are quite challenging to orient oneself, for the simple reason that they are performed from below upwards almost like an upside-down surgery. Writing on a subject of this kind requires a vast amount of expertise and experience in handling a variety of cases, including the complicated ones.

This book has made a difficult subject ridiculously simple. There is no aspect of the subject that is untouched and undescribed. The book is well-planned, and the chapters are neatly organized to amicably address even the minutest detail on the subject.

This book is very useful for students for their exams, as well as for other practitioners in skull base surgery to treat day-to-day cases in common events like road traffic accidents.

I wish this book a great success and recommend it to all the students and practitioners of ENT, skull base surgery, and neurosurgery to master the skills of these challenging procedures.

Vikram K Bhat MS, DNB, MNAMS, PhD (ENT)
Professor and Unit Chief
Department of Otorhinolaryngology – Head and Neck Surgery
Karnataka Institute of Medical Sciences
Hubli, Karnataka, India

## COMPREHENSIVE, SYSTEMATIC, PRECISE

These are the three words that came to mind when I first read this book from Dr Jyotirmay Hegde. Whilst CSF rhinorrhea is a familiar topic to most ENT and neurosurgeons, there is much to learn from this book. Initially, the repairs were transcranial or transfacial, but as nasal endoscopy spread its wings, we discovered the potential of endoscopic endonasal surgery. Even though most repairs are done endoscopically today, the young surgeon still faces some apprehension. This is sometimes due to the location, maybe the size, or the intracranial pressure, but usually the fear of failing. Having explained the risk of meningitis to convince the patient of the need for surgery, one does want to ensure the correct approach and technique to ensure a good closure. The information given here about CSF rhinorrhea and its management will be valuable in your quest to attain perfect results.

Dr Hegde has done an extremely good job in writing and organizing this book in a way that encompasses the various aspects in a lucid manner. It starts with an interesting chapter on the history of CSF leaks, before going on to the physiology. He then gives us a few chapters on classification and etiology before getting to the business end of surgical repair. These include details of techniques with some wonderful photos and videos, including those for skull base reconstruction. The book also incorporates radiology and complications to ensure that we truly have a complete compilation and knowledge of CSF leaks.

Dr Jyotirmay Hegde came to me as a young clinical fellow in 2009, very eager to learn endoscopic skull base surgery. He has traveled a long road since then, and it certainly is a proud moment for a teacher to see his young student become one of India's shining stars in endoscopic sinus and skull base surgery.

I feel privileged to write this foreword for Dr Hegde and recommend it as a wonderful resource for all rhinologists – both young and experienced.

Dr Nishit Shah
Senior ENT Consultant
Bombay Hospital and Breach Candy Hospital
Mumbai, India

# CLEAR, LOGICAL, AND PRACTICAL APPROACH TO THE COMPLETE TOPIC

It gives me great pleasure to write a foreword for this unique book that comprehensively covers a topic that holds so much fascination. Cerebrospinal rhinorrhea from the anterior skull base continues to challenge many rhinologists and will always generate much opinion, controversy, and discussion. The list of 15 chapters offers a clear, logical, ordered, and practical approach to the complete topic. These are supplemented by clear diagrams and an excellent range of scans and superb peri-operative images.

The book deals initially with a description of the historical aspects of CSF rhinorrhea. Several decades ago, attempting endonasal surgery to stop CSF rhinorrhoea was said to be too dangerous and that such management should be avoided. This led to the long-held concept that since most CSF leaks eventually stop, the preferred management was conservative with bed rest and medication, and surgery was reserved for intransigent cases.

The risk element of intracranial infection and particularly meningitis with remaining skull base defects was not fully appreciated for many years, and the true incidence of intracranial complications only became apparent about 30 years ago.

This coincided with the development of extended approaches of endoscopic sinus surgery, enabling safe access to the anterior skull base. In parallel to the latter, there were huge improvements in radiological imaging techniques. It therefore became possible to not only identify and localize the source of the leak, but also to gain access and repair the skull base defect.

It soon became apparent that most cases could be performed endonasally and endoscopically. On occasions, these techniques were combined with external approaches, particularly for frontal sinus leaks. The need for craniotomy and intracranial repair therefore became much reduced. Whilst this change offered a huge advantage to patients with a lower morbidity, preservation in the sense of smell, and short hospital stay, it demanded surgeons learn new skills, and there was less opportunity for neurosurgeons to learn and practice intracranial repair. New skills were soon discovered, particularly with regard to techniques of the repair and the advantages of multi-layered repair and the use of locally-based vascularised flaps.

This textbook thus brings all surgical aspects of intracranial, external, endoscopic and endonasal repair together, maintaining an important balance in knowledge and learning.

The book also offers clear guidance on important basic information such as radiological imaging techniques, the use of intrathecal fluorescein to locate the skull base defect, as well as the subtleties in management that generate so much discussion. A dedicated textbook that collates the various aspects of this disorder will therefore prove to be a valuable asset to all who read it.

Andrew C. Swift ChM, FRCS, FRCS(Ed)
Consultant Rhinologist and ENT Surgeon
Aintree University Hospital, Liverpool
Honorary Senior Lecturer
University of Liverpool and Edge Hill University
President-elect ENT UK

# Preface

Cerebrospinal fluid (CSF) rhinorrhea is a potentially devastating condition that can lead to significant morbidity and mortality for the patient. The communication between the central nervous system (CNS) and the sinonasal cavity can result in a multitude of infectious complications that impart significant morbidity and potentially disastrous long-term deficits for the patient. From the first intracranial repair in the 1900s to the use of endoscopes and image-guidance systems, the management of CSF rhinorrhea has greatly evolved. Dandy is credited with the first surgical repair of a CSF leak via a frontal craniotomy approach in 1926. Various other authors, including Dohlman (1948), Hirsch (1952), and Hallberg (1964), subsequently reported successful repair of CSF rhinorrhea through different external approaches. In 1981, Wigand reported on the use of the endoscope to assist with the repair of a skull base defect. Since then, endoscopic repair has become the preferred method of addressing CSF rhinorrhea, given the high success rate of 90–95% and the decreased morbidity associated with this approach.

The need for writing this book is to provide a comprehensive approach in the management and practice of CSF rhinorrhea. What makes this book stand out is the exclusive manner in which it is written. We have made a point to cover all the aspects of CSF rhinorrhea yet keeping it concise and precise. This book covers from the history of CSF rhinorrhea to basic aspects of CSF production, diagnosis of leak to both transcranial and endoscopic management of CSF rhinorrhea. The various causes of CSF rhinorrhea such as traumatic, idiopathic, and iatrogenic events have been explained in detail. Systemic causes of CSF rhinorrhea and management of benign intracranial hypertension has been dealt elaborately. We have also included an exclusive chapter to showcase the role of navigation in the management of CSF leaks. It also provides a detailed description of the various techniques used in the reconstruction of skull-base defects to the recent advances in the field of CSF rhinorrhea. The combination of text, figures, flowcharts, and video clips should give the reader confidence to tackle various technical challenges that can occur during the surgery.

We hope that the book will be an important resource in the field of CSF rhinorrhea for undergraduates, postgraduates in otorhinolaryngology, neurosurgery, neuromedicine, radiology, and internal medicine, and for practicing clinicians, surgeons, radiologists, and budding rhinologists.

# Acknowledgments

This book has been possible because of the guidance of my beloved teachers who have been instrumental in shaping my career and helping me to become what I am. I would like to thank all my teachers who have been the guiding force behind this book. However, I would especially thank the three musketeers in my life, Dr Vikram Bhat, Dr Nishit Shah, and Mr Andrew Swift, whom I owe for everything they have taught me in the field of endoscopic sinus and skull-base surgery. I am very grateful to them for writing the foreword for this book.

I must also acknowledge and thank my co-author Dr Hemanth Vamanshankar, for his dedication and perseverance. He has spent endless hours and days working tirelessly, and this endeavor would not have been possible without his efforts. He is not only an excellent clinician but a wonderful colleague as well.

I must also thank the entire administrative and hospital staff at Columbia Asia Hospital, Whitefield, Bangalore for their help and support in pursuing my passion. A special thanks to Dr Nandakumar Jairam, Chairman and CEO, Columbia Asia Hospitals, India, for his constant motivation and encouragement, and I owe him a huge debt of gratitude. I would also like to thank my ENT and neurosurgical colleagues at Columbia Asia Hospital and former colleagues with whom I have been fortunate to work with at SDM Medical College, Dharwad and JIPMER, Pondicherry.

I would like to thank my family for always encouraging, pushing me forward, and raising the bar higher in constant pursuit of excellence. My parents Dr Shyamsundar V Hegde and Mrs Veena Hegde for their patience and understanding and for nurturing in me the values required to live in peace and happiness. My brother Tanmay for always being there with me. My wife, Shreshta, and my loving kids Anurag and Arna from whom I have received encouragement, fortitude, and love.

I would also like to thank Ms Shivangi Pramanik and Himani Dwivedi from CRC Press, Taylor & Francis, for having confidence in me and their constant support. Last but not least, I would like to thank my patients without whom this book would not have materialized.

I will always be indebted to the almighty and loving God for giving me the strength, guidance, and perseverance to complete this task.

Jyotirmay S Hegde

# Editors

## DR JYOTIRMAY S HEGDE

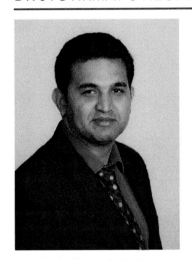

**Dr Jyotirmay S Hegde** is a Consulting ENT, Head and Neck & Endoscopic skull base surgeon at Columbia Asia Hospital, Whitefield, Bangalore.

He completed his Masters in Otolaryngology – Head & Neck Surgery at Karnataka Institute of Medical Sciences, Hubli, Karnataka (India). He has worked as a faculty member in various capacities at Jawaharlal Institute of Postgraduate Medical Education & Research (JIPMER), Pondicherry, India. He is a Fellow of the European Board of Otolaryngology (FEBORL). He also completed his Fellowship in Rhinology and Endoscopic skull-base surgery from University Hospital Aintree, Liverpool, UK. He also completed his fellowship in Endoscopic sinus surgery at Bombay Hospital, Mumbai, India. He was awarded the Cipla fellowship award for the best outgoing student during his Masters. He is the recipient of the prestigious Dr P. N. Berry fellowship and was awarded the British Annual Congress in Otolaryngology (BACO) fellowship during 2015 and the International visiting scholarship at the American Academy of Otolaryngology Head & Neck Surgery at Chicago in 2017. He has also been a recipient of the travelling fellowship by the German Society of Otolaryngology, Head and Neck Surgery in 2017. He received a gold medal for the best video presentation at AOICON, Kolkata, India and has published in several peer-reviewed scientific publications and presented at national and international conferences, courses, and workshops.

# DR HEMANTH VAMANSHANKAR

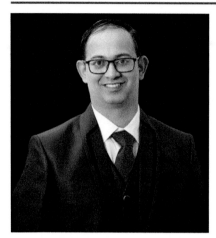

**Dr Hemanth Vamanshankar** graduated from K. S. Hegde Medical Academy, Mangalore in 2008, and completed a Diploma in Otolaryngology from St John's Medical College, Bangalore in 2011, and DNB-ENT from Railway Hospital, Ayanavaram, Chennai in 2014. He was awarded an MRCS-ENT from the Royal College of Surgeons, Edinburgh. He has to his credit 25 indexed publications of national and international repute. He is currently working as a medical officer and Consultant ENT Surgeon at the Divisional Railway Hospital, Bangalore (South Western Railway).

# List of contributors

**Shreshta Bhat**
Prima Diagnostics
Columbia Asia Hospital
Bengaluru, Karnataka, India

**Harsh Deora**
Department of Neurosurgery
National Institute of Mental Health
and Neurosciences (NIMHANS)
Bengaluru, Karnataka, India

**Mohammed Nadeem**
Department of Neurosurgery
National Institute of Mental Health
and Neurosciences (NIMHANS)
Bengaluru, Karnataka, India

**Nishant Sadashiva**
Department of Neurosurgery
National Institute of Mental Health
and Neurosciences (NIMHANS)
Bengaluru, Karnataka, India

# History of CSF rhinorrhea

## HEMANTH VAMANSHANKAR AND JYOTIRMAY S HEGDE

St Clair Thomson, a British surgeon and professor of laryngology, gave the first description of a CSF rhinorrhea following a skull fracture in 1899[1] (Figure 1.1). The first description of a spontaneous CSF leak was given by Charles Miller.[2] In 1884, after a post mortem, Chiari incidentally discovered a communication of the brain with the ethmoids, with the presence of an aerocele in one of his patients.[3] Although these were merely clinical diagnoses, the first radiological description of an aerocele performed by X-ray technique was given by Luckett in 1913.[4]

Walter Edward Dandy, considered one of the founding fathers of neurosurgery from Johns Hopkins University (Figure 1.2), is credited as the first person to undertake an external CSF leak repair through a bifrontal craniotomy in 1926[5] (the fascia lata was used to plug a leak in the posterior wall of the frontal sinus). This continued to be the treatment of choice until Dohlman in 1948, who described the extracranial naso-orbital incision used in order to repair an anterior cranial fossa leak.[6] An unsuccessful attempt of leak repair for a traumatic aerocele was performed by Grant in 1923.[7] A transnasal approach to sphenoid sinus leaks using septal flaps was reported by Hirsch in 1952.[8] An intranasal approach for cribriform plate leaks was described by Vrabec and Hallberg in 1964.[9] The use of endoscopes for the repair of small CSF leaks occurring during ethmoidectomy began only in 1981, popularized by Wigand.[10]

For closure of CSF leaks, fascia lata was the primary choice, as described by Dandy. This was similarly described by others like Cushing (1927), McKinney (1932), Cairns (1937), Gissane and Rank (1940), Eden (1942), and Campbell, Howard, and Weary (1942).[11–16] Echols and Holcombe (1941)[17] described closure by using muscle. German (1944)[18] described using flaps of dura covering the crista galli and falx to repair five cases. The use of a free periosteal graft over the cribriform plate was described by Ecker in 1947.[19] The use of absorbable gelatin sponge (Gelfoam) was first mentioned by Cloward and Cunningham in 1947.[20] The use of wax after stripping the dura on either side of the CSF leak and subsequent

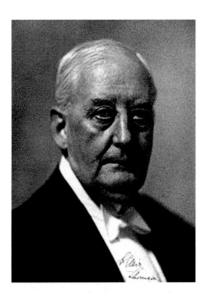

Figure 1.1 St Clair Thomson (1859–1943). © Jyotirmay S Hegde, Hemanth Vamanshankar.

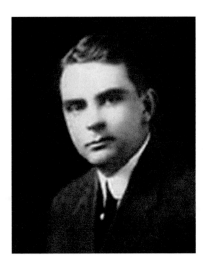

Figure 1.2 Walter Edward Dandy (1886–1946). © Jyotirmay S Hegde, Hemanth Vamanshankar.

suturing was successfully described by Love and Gay.[21] Coleman described the release of air and suturing dura over cribriform plate – which he successfully performed in a case of pneumatocele with CSF rhinorrhea following trauma.[22]

It is, however, interesting to note the other anecdotal forms of treatment used for CSF leaks.

50% chromic acid has been used for cauterizing the CSF, which had been said to cure a CSF leak by B. de Almeida.[23]

Lumbar puncture, attempted during an episode of meningitis, is said to have stopped a CSF leak, as described by Singleton.[24] Similar cases were described by Schroeder and Frenzel (who along with lumbar puncture also started the patient on sulfonamides).[25,26]

Radiation has also been described as a possible cure for CSF leaks, with Sgalitzer describing cure in nine out of ten patients.[27] This he ascribed to the fact that X-ray irradiation to the choroid plexus causes inhibition of CSF production, and hence halts the leaks.

Learmouth is said to have inserted cotton packs soaked in tincture of iodine extradurally over the cribriform plate for nine days, causing a cessation of drainage.[28]

## REFERENCES

1. Thomson St. C. *The Cerebro-Spinal Fluid: Its Spontaneous Escape from the Nose.* London, UK: Cassell & Co., Ltd., 1899, p. 8.
2. Thomson S and Negus VE. *Diseases of the Nose and Throat* (5th edition). New York: Appleton-Century-Crofts, Inc., 1947, p. 104.
3. Chiari H. Ueber einen Fall von Luftansammlung in den Ventrikeln des menschlichen Gehirns. *Ztschr f Heilk* 5:383, 1884.
4. Luckett WH. Air in the ventricle of the brain following fracture of the skull. *Surgery, Gynecology & Obstetrics* 17:237, 1913.
5. Dandy WE. Pneumocephalus (Internal pneumocele or aeroscele). *Archives of Surgery* 12:949–982, 1926.
6. Dohlman G. Spontaneous cerebrospinal rhinorrhea. *Acta Otorrinolaringologica* 67:20–23, 1948.
7. Grant FC. Intracranial aerocele following a fracture of the skull. *Surgery, Gynecology & Obstetrics* 36:251, 1923.
8. Lanza DC, O'Brien DA and Kennedy DW. *Endoscopic repair of cerebrospinal fluid fistulae and encephaloceles.* Laryngoscope 106:1119–1125, 1996.
9. Vrabec DP, Hallberg OE. Cerebrospinal fluid rhinorrhea. *Archives of Otolaryngology* 80:218–229, 1964.
10. Wigand WE. Transnasal ethmoidectomy under endoscopic control. *Rhinology* 19:7–15, 1981.
11. Cushing H. Experiences with orbito-ethmoidal osteomata having intracranial complications, with the report of four cases, *Surgery, Gynecology & Obstetrics* 44:721–742, 1927.
12. McKinney R. Traumatic pneumocephalus. *The Annals of Otology, Rhinology, and Laryngology* 41:597–600, 1932.
13. Cairns H. Injuries of the frontal and ethmoidal sinuses with special reference to cerebro-spinal rhinorrhoea and aeroceles. *The Journal of Laryngology and Otology* 52:589–623, 1937.

14. Gissane W and Rank BK. Post-Traumatic cerebro-spinal rhinorrhoea with case report. *British Journal of Surgery* 27:717, 1940.
15. Eden K. Traumatic cerebro-spinal rhinorrhoea: Repair of a fistula by a transfrontal intradural operation. *British Journal of Surgery* 29:299–303, 1942.
16. Campbell E, Howard WP and Weary WB. Gunshot wounds of the brain. *Archives of Surgery* 44:789, 1942.
17. Echols DH and Holcombe RG. Traumatic intra-cerebral pneumatocele. *Southern Surgeon* 10:589–591, 1941.
18. German WG. Cerebro-spinal rhinorrhea-surgical repair. *Journal of Neurosurgery* 1:60–66, 1944.
19. Ecker A. Cerebro-spinal rhinorrhea by way of the eustachian tube. *Journal of Neurosurgery* 4:177–180, 1947.
20. Cloward RB and Cunningham BE. The use of gelatine sponge in prevention and treatment of cerebro-spinal rhinorrhea. *Journal of Neurosurgery* 4:519–525, 1947.
21. Love GJ and Gay JR. Spontaneous cerebro-spinal rhinorrhea: Successful surgical treatment. *Archives of Otolaryngology* 46:40–44, 1947.
22. Coleman CC. Fracture of the skull involving paranasal sinuses and mastoids. *JAMA* 109:1613–1616, 1937.
23. de Almeida B. Zwei Fälle von Kranio-rhinorrhoe. *Monatsschr Ohrenh* 62:322–326, 1928.
24. Singleton AB. Leakage of cerebro-spinal fluid through cribriform plate of ethmoid bone. *Canadian Medical Association Journal* 24:838–839, 1931.
25. Schroeder MC. Meningitis due to posttraumatic cerebro-spinal rhinorrhea. *Archives of Otolaryngology* 40:206–207, 1944.
26. Frenzel. Discussion. *Monatsschr Ohrenh* 185:43, 1951.
27. Sgalitzer M. Erfahrungen mit der Roentgenbehandlung von Liquorfisteln, Wien. med. *Wchnschr* 80:1195–1197, 1930.
28. Learmouth JR. Cerebro-spinal rhinorrhea treated by operation. *Proceedings of the Staff Meetings of the Mayo Clinic* 4:115, 1929.

# 2

# Basics of CSF production

## HEMANTH VAMANSHANKAR AND JYOTIRMAY S HEGDE

Hippocrates first discussed CSF as water surrounding the brain while describing congenital hydrocephalus. However, the discovery of CSF is credited to the Swedish philosopher and scientist, Emanuel Swedenborg, who in his manuscript written in the early 18th century, described CSF as a "spiritous lymph" produced in the fourth ventricle and going down into the spinal cord. CSF is formed in the cerebral ventricles – mainly the choroid plexus, ependyma, and parenchyma.[1] Produced at the rate of 500 mL/day or 03–0.4 mL/min, a total of 90–150 mL volume is present in an adult. Of this total, 25% is present in the ventricular system (35 mL), 20–50% is present in the spinal canal (30–70 mL) and about 25–55% is to be found in the cranial subarachnoid space (35–75 mL).[2,3] Out of the 1600–1700 ml intracranial space which encloses the brain, about 100–150 mL is occupied by the CSF. But, interestingly, this small volume of CSF has the capacity to reduce the actual weight of the brain (1500 gm) to as much as 50 mg, hence reducing the risk of brain injury, as well as tension on nerve roots and vessels.[4–8]

CSF (and to a lesser extent blood) is the primary buffer whose volume decreases in compensation to an increase in intracranial volume – according to the Monro-Kellie doctrine.[2,3]

CSF has a mean production of 0.36 ml/min and a density of 1.003–1.008 g/cm.[9] Beta-2-transferrin, being specific to CSF (found otherwise only in perilymph and ocular fluids) is a desialated isoform of the iron-binding glycoprotein transferrin.[10] β-trace protein (βTP), the second most abundant protein in human CSF after albumin and produced in epithelial cells of the choroid plexus, is another potential marker of CSF diagnosis. It is thought to be important in the maturation and maintenance of CSF as it is identical to prostaglandin D synthase. It also has a higher sensitivity and specificity as a CSF marker than β2 transferrin. Chemically, CSF has a higher concentration of chloride and lower concentrations of potassium, protein and glucose, as compared to plasma.[11]

Functionally the CSF acts as a protective cushion to the brain and spinal cord; it acts as a lymphatic system; and also has roles in chemical buffering, neurodevelopment, homeostatic hormonal and signaling mechanisms.[5,12–16] CSF is also involved in the supply and distribution of growth factors like IGF-2, TGF, GH, FGF and arginine vasopressin. It also acts to eliminate xenobiotics and endogenous waste from CSF to blood.[4,14,17,18]

The choroid plexus is present in the 3rd and 4th ventricle roof, and walls of the lateral ventricle. The plexus, responsible for 60–70% CSF production, has a rich blood supply – ten times that of the cortex – from the anterior choroidal, lateral posterior choroidal, paired medial posterior choroidal and posterior inferior cerebellar arteries.[9] Venous networks coalesce to form a single large vein. The epithelium is lined by simple cuboidal cells with cilia having a large surface area of approximately 200 cm$^2$.[5] The exchange of solutes and fluids is controlled by barriers in the epithelium of the choroid plexus. These include metabolic barriers, i.e. apical brush border-expressing peptidases; cellular barriers based on transporter proteins that are membrane specific; and mechanical barriers, i.e. tight junctions.[5,6,16,19,20]

The walls of ventricles are composed of specialized cells, tanycytes, which are scattered among the ependymal cells. They are believed to regulate neuroendocrine function.[21,22] The basement membrane beneath the ependymal layer forms labyrinths, which connect to the subependymal basement membrane capillaries and veins. These have the capacity to hold fluid in them by swelling.[23]

CSF production is controlled within the epithelium by membrane transporters. The leaky vascular endothelial wall of the choroid plexus epithelial cells allows ultrafiltration of solutes, ions and water from plasma. At the apical (CSF-facing) membranes is present a K+/Cl – a cotransporter with Na+/K+ -ATPase and also a high AQP1 expression – which together expel water from the cell into the CSF space.[24]

CSF secretion: From formation in the lateral and third ventricles – to its flow through the foramen of Monro and aqueduct of Sylvius; leaving the fourth ventricle through the foramen of Magendie and foramina of Lushka – CSF gets absorbed into the blood at arachnoid villi on the superior sagittal sinus. In the spinal canal, CSF spaces extend right from the foramen magnum to filum terminale, surrounding the nerve roots and spinal cord. The arachnoid villi are invaginations of the arachnoid into the venous area. These are present in the regions of arachnoid angles in spinal roots and cranial venous sinuses. Pacchionian or arachnoid granulations are formed when there is a massive dilatation of the subarachnoid space within a villus, named after Pacchioni, who first described them in 1721. Granulations, however, form from the age of 18 months in humans (Figure 2.1 A, B). Recent studies using 3D MRI techniques have shown the majority of granulations are situated at the superior sagittal (54%), transverse (28%) and straight sinus (18%).[25–27] This entire circulation of CSF is termed the "third circulation".[1]

The subarachnoid space is comprised of two layers: an outer barrier cell layer and an inner trabecular layer. The trabecular layer has extracellular collagen, and forms cisterns of various shapes and sizes, through which nerves and vessels

## ANATOMY OF ARACHNOID GRANULATION

(A)                                         (B)

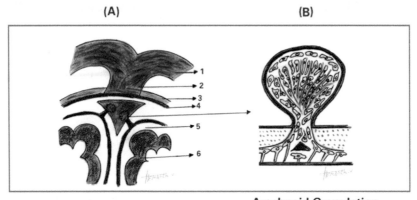

1. Transverse Sinus
2. Superior Sagittal Sinus
3. Dura
4. Arachnoid
5. CSF
6. Brain Parenchyma

Arachnoid Granulation

Figure 2.1 (A, B): Anatomy of arachnoid granulation. © Jyotirmay S Hegde, Hemanth Vamanshankar.

traverse. CSF normally flows through these cisterns. Communicating hydro-cephalus develops due to the obstruction of the flow of CSF through these cis-terns[28,29] (Figure 2.2 A).

Reabsorption also takes place over lymphatics across the cribriform plate (extra-arachnoidal cranical CSF clearance route)[30] and nerve root subarachnoid angles.[9] CSF drainage through spinal lymphatic routes has also been proposed. Healthy human volunteers were tested using radionucleotides, and found to have 0.11–0.23 mL/min absorption of CSF through these spinal routes, which increased during exercise.[31]

Flow through the ventricles is in a pulsatile manner, the flow being influ-enced by movements of spinal cord and brain with respiration and cardiac sys-tole, movement of ependymal cilia and pressure gradients between subarachnoid space, venous and lymphatic spaces.[9] This is further explained by the Windkessel effect of CSF drainage. The systolic phase of blood pressure causes arterial disten-sion, while the diastolic phase causes arterial recoiling. The energy thus produced is transferred to the brain as CSF and brain pulsations. This pulsatile flow kinetic energy is said to be 100 fold greater than bulk flow kinetic energy. This energy however dissipates, while maintaining a low intracranial pressure, which in turn provides for a high cerebral blood flow.[32]

More important than the conventional pathway is the flow of CSF through the Virchow-Robin spaces (VRS), which are involved in cerebral water movement. These are spaces histologically surrounding blood vessels as CSF moves from a subarachnoid space into brain tissue. VRS is a complex formed by the endothelial, pial, and glial cell layers, thus allowing a bidirectional fluid exchange. At the regions of the capillaries, the basement membranes of the glia and endothelium join, thus obliterating the VRS (Figure 2.2 A–C). The presence of VRS has been demonstrated experimentally by numerous tracers like horseradish peroxidase, India ink, albumin labeled with colloidal gold, Evans blue, and rhodamine.[33,34]

Transport of water, solutes, and ions in a bi-directional manner, in response to both hydraulic pressure and passive osmotic gradients, is controlled by aquaporins. These are highly selective of the molecule being transported, and at the same time provide rapid transport.[35] Of the many aquaporins found (about 14 are identified), six are reported to be present in the brain.[36-38] Permeability is specific to each of them; AQP3 and 9- permeable to small solutes and water; AQP8 to ions; and AQP 1, 4, 5 are water permeable. Of these, AQP1 is important in CSF formation; AQP9 in energy metabolism; AQP4 in the clearance of K+ released in neuronal activity and formation/resolution of brain edema.[36] AQP4 channels move water by simple diffusion and vesicular transport – this is currently the most accepted theory of the function of AQP4 (Figure 2.2 C).[39] Further, AQP4-rich areas like BBB and glia limitans at the subpial zones may also act as water channels for ISF-CSF drainage in extreme conditions.[40] The discovery of aquaporins by Peter Agre, which resulted in his receiving a Nobel Prize in Chemistry

## ANATOMY OF CSF PATHWAY & VIRCHOW-ROBIN SPACES

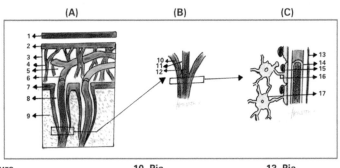

| 1. Dura | 10. Pia | 13. Pia |
|---|---|---|
| 2. Arachnoid | 11. VRS | 14. Capillary |
| 3. Sub-arachnoid space | 12. Capillary | 15. AQP4 at glia limitans |
| 4. Arachnoid trabeculae | | 16. Tight junctions |
| 5. Cisterns | * At Capillary end, the | 17. Astrocytes in |
| 6. Blood Vessels | VRS is obliterated as the | brain parenchyma |
| 7. Pia | glial & endothelial | |
| 8. Virchow-Robin space (VRS) | basemembranes join | |
| 9. Brain parenchyma | | |

Figure 2.2 (A, B, C): Anatomy of CSF pathway and Virchow-Robin spaces. © Jyotirmay S Hegde, Hemanth Vamanshankar.

in 2003, has led us to a greater understanding of biological fluid homeostasis and turnover.[41]

## TAKE-HOME POINTS

- CSF is produced at a rate of 500 mL/day with a total volume of 90–150 mL in an adult.
- B trace protein is now considered a better sensitive and specific marker than β2 transferrin in CSF identification.
- CSF flow through ventricles, contributing to the maintenance of low intracranial pressure and high cerebral blood flow, as explained by the Windkessel effect.
- Virchow-Robin spaces have an important function in cerebral water movement.
- The transport of water and solutes in CSF is contributed by aquaporins.

## REFERENCES

1. McComb JG. Recent research into the nature of cerebrospinal fluid formation and absorption. *J Neurosurg* 1983; 59: 369–83.
2. Kohn MI, Tanna NK, Herman GT et al. Analysis of brain and cerebrospinal fluid volumes with MR imaging. Part I. Methods, reliability, and validation. *Radiology* 1991; 178 (1): 115–22.
3. Redzic ZB, Segal MB. The structure of the choroid plexus and the physiology of the choroid plexus epithelium. *Adv Drug Delivery Rev* 2004; 56 (12): 1695–716.
4. Hall GA. *Medical Physiology* (11th edition). Philadelphia, PA: Elsevier Saunders, 2006.
5. Kimelberg HK. Water homeostasis in the brain: Basic concepts. *Neuroscience* 2004; 129 (4): 851–60.
6. Redzic ZB, Preston JE, Duncan JA, Chodobski A, Szmydynger-Chodobska J. The choroid plexus cerebrospinal fluid system: From development to aging. *Curr Top Dev Biol* 2005; 71: 1–52.
7. Chodobski A, Szmydynger-Chodobska J. Choroid plexus: Target for polypeptides and site of their synthesis. *Microsc Res Tech* 2001; 52 (1): 65–82.
8. Oldendorf WH, Davson H. Brain extracellular space and the sink action of cerebrospinal fluid. Measurement of rabbit brain extracellular space using sucrose labelled with carbon 14. *Arch Neurol* 1967; 17 (2): 196–205.
9. Davson H, Segal MB. *Physiology of the CSF and Blood Brain Barriers*. Boca Raton, FL: CRC Press, 1996.
10. Papadea C, Schlosser RJ. Rapid method for beta2-transferrin in cerebrospinal fluid leakage using an automated immunofixation electrophoresis system. *Clin Chem* 2005; 51: 464–70.

11. Johanson CE, Stopa EG, McMillan PN. The blood cerebrospinal fluid barrier: Structure and functional significance. *Methods Mol Biol* 2011; 686: 101–31.
12. Redzic ZB, Segal MB. The structure of the choroid plexus and the physiology of the choroid plexus epithelium. *Adv Drug Delivery Rev* 2004; 56: 1695–716.
13. Rosenberg GA. *Brain Fluids and Metabolism*. Oxford, UK: Oxford University Press, 1990.
14. Miaki K, Matsui H, Nakano M, Tsuji H. Nutritional supply to the cauda equina in lumbar adhesive arachnoiditis in rats. *Eur Spine J* 1999; 8 (4): 310–16.
15. Brown PD, Davies SL, Speake T, Millar ID. Molecular mechanisms of cerebrospinal fluid production. *Neuroscience* 2004; 129: 957–70.
16. Jones HC. Cerebrospinal fluid research: A new platform for dissemination of research, opinions and reviews with a common theme. *Cerebrospinal Fluid Res* 2004; 1: 1.
17. Smith DE, Johanson CE, Keep RF. Peptide and peptide analog transport systems at the blood-CSF barrier. *Adv Drug Delivery Rev* 2004; 56: 1765–91.
18. Emerich DF, Skinner SJ, Borlongan CV, Vasconcellos AV, Thanos CG. The choroid plexus in the rise, fall and repair of the brain. *Bioessays* 2005; 27 (3): 262–74.
19. Kusuhara H, Sugiyama Y. Efflux transport systems for organic anions and cations at the blood – CSF barrier. *Adv Drug Delivery Rev* 2004; 56: 1741–63.
20. Vorbrodt AW, Dobrogowska DH. Molecular anatomy of interendothelial junctions in human blood – brain barrier microvessels. *Folia Histochem Cytobiol* 2004; 42 (2): 67–75.
21. Wittkowski W. Tanycytes and pituicytes: Morphological and functional aspects of neuroglial interaction. *Microsc Res Tech* 1998; 41 (1): 29–42.
22. Rodriguez EM, Blázquez JL, Pastor FE et al. Hypothalamic tanycytes: A key component of brain endocrine interaction. *Int Rev Cytol* 2005; 247: 89–164.
23. Leonhardt H, Desaga U. Recent observations on ependyma and subependymal basement membranes. *Acta Neurochir* 1975; 31 (3–4): 153–9.
24. Praetorius J, Nielsen S. Distribution of sodium transporters and aquaporin-1 in the human choroid plexus. *Am J Physiol Cell Physiol* 2006; 291: C59–67.
25. Williams PL, Warwick R, Dyson M, Bannister LH (Eds.). *Gray's Anatomy* (37th edition). London, UK: Churchill Livingstone, 1989.
26. Weed LH. The pathways of escape from the subarachnoid spaces with particular reference to the arachnoid villi. *J Med Res* 1914; 31: 51–91.
27. Liang L, Korogi Y, Sugahara T et al. Normal structures in the intracranial dural sinuses: Delineation with 3D contrast enhanced magnetization prepared rapid acquisition gradient echo imaging sequence. *Am J Neuroradiol* 2002; 23: 1739–46.

28. Haines DE. On the question of a subdural space. *Anat Rec* 1991; 230 (1): 3–21.
29. Li J, McAllister JP 2nd, Shen Y et al. Communicating hydrocephalus in adult rats with kaolin obstruction of the basal cisterns or the cortical subarachnoid space. *Exp Neurol* 2008; 211 (2): 351–61.
30. Koh L, Zakharov A, Johnston M. Integration of the subarachnoid space and lymphatics: Is it time to embrace a new concept of cerebrospinal fluid absorption? *Cerebrospinal Fluid Res* 2005; 2 (1): 6.
31. Edsbagge M, Starck G, Zetterberg H, Ziegelitz D, Wikkelso C. Spinal cerebrospinal fluid volume in healthy elderly individuals. *Clin Anat* 2011; 24 (6): 733–40.
32. Min KJ, Yoon SH, Kang JK. New understanding of the role of cerebrospinal fluid: Offsetting of arterial and brain pulsation and self-dissipation of cerebrospinal fluid pulsatile flow energy. *Med Hypotheses* 2011; 76 (6): 884–6.
33. Ichimura T, Fraser PA, Cserr HF. Distribution of extracellular tracers in perivascular spaces of the rat brain. *Brain Res* 1991; 545: 103–13.
34. Rennels ML, Gregory TF, Blaumanis OR, Fujimoto K, Grady PA. Evidence for a 'paravascular' fluid circulation in the mammalian central nervous system, provided by the rapid distribution of tracer protein throughout the brain from the subarachnoid space. *Brain Res* 1985; 326: 47–63.
35. Agre P. The aquaporin water channels. *Proc Am Thorac Soc* 2006; 3: 5–13.
36. Papadopoulos MC, Verkman AS. Aquaporin water channels in the nervous system. *Nat Rev Neurosci* 2013; 14: 265–77.
37. Chai RC, Jiang JH, Kwan Wong AY et al. AQP5 is differentially regulated in astrocytes during metabolic and traumatic injuries. *Glia* 2013; 61: 1748–65.
38. Igarashi H, Tsujita M, Kwee IL, Nakada T. Water influx into cerebrospinal fluid is primarily controlled by aquaporin-4, not by aquaporin-1: 17O JJVCPE MRI study in knockout mice. *Neuroreport* 2014; 25 (1): 39–43.
39. Tait MJ, Saadoun S, Bell BA, Papadopoulos MC. Water movements in the brain: Role of aquaporins. *Trends Neurosci* 2008; 31: 37–43.
40. Bloch O, Auguste KI, Manley GT, Verkman AS. Accelerated progression of kaolin-induced hydrocephalus in aquaporin-4-dei cient mice. *J Cerebral Blood Flow Metab* 2006; 26 (12): 1527–37.
41. Agre P, Nielsen S, Ottersen OP. Towards a molecular understanding of water homeostasis in the brain. *Neuroscience* 2004; 129 (4): 849–50.

# 3

# Classification of CSF rhinorrhea

HEMANTH VAMANSHANKAR AND JYOTIRMAY S HEGDE

In 1937, Cairns, a British neurosurgeon, developed the first classification system for CSF rhinorrhea and proposed the following subtypes: acute traumatic, delayed traumatic, spontaneous, and postoperative.[1] O'Connell, in 1964, further subclassified spontaneous leaks into idiopathic or primary types, wherein a cause could not be found, and into secondary types.[2] In 1968, Ommaya redefined the classification given by O'Connell (Figure 3.1).[3]

Various types of classifications of CSF rhinorrhea are presented here. Leaks can present from the anterior, middle, or posterior cranial fossa (Figure 3.2). The majority of leaks in the middle or posterior cranial fossa present into the nose through the Eustachian tube. However, in cases where there is extensive pneumatisation of the sphenoid sinus laterally or petrous bone medial pneumatisation, leaks originating in the temporal bone can travel via petrous apex and sphenoid sinus into the nose.[4]

Traumatic leaks may present early as an acute leak or have a delayed presentation. They are classified based on the most common site of occurrence of the leak following trauma (Figure 3.3). A careful examination of the patient's history in cases of spontaneous leaks may sometimes point to a delayed traumatic leak – some which may have occurred many years ago.[5,6]

Spontaneous leaks may be further classified into high pressure and normal pressure leaks (Figure 3.4). It is essential to first treat the pathological process in cases of high-pressure leak before a formal closure of the leak is attempted, as otherwise a failure is imminent. The concept of "focal atrophy" has been explained by Ommaya et al. as a cause of a normal pressure leak. They explained that due to ischemia and secondary loss of tissue bulk in regions of the cribriform plate and

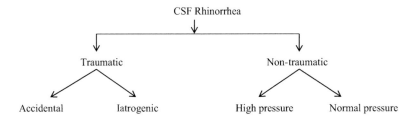

Figure 3.1 Original classification of CSF leaks by Ommaya et al. © Jyotirmay S Hegde, Hemanth Vamanshankar.

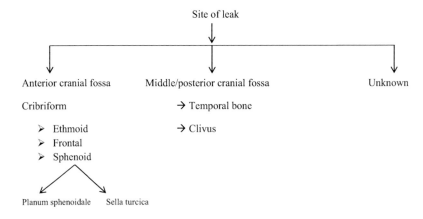

Figure 3.2 Classification of CSF leaks: based on site of leak. © Jyotirmay S Hegde, Hemanth Vamanshankar.

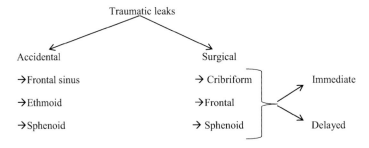

Figure 3.3 Classification of CSF leaks: traumatic leaks. © Jyotirmay S Hegde, Hemanth Vamanshankar.

sella turcica, there was a formation of pulsatile arachnoid pouches which erode the underlying bone. Eventually, a fistula with or without a meningoencephalocele may form, and result in a further CSF leak.

Idiopathic CSF rhinorrhea is extremely rare (Figure 3.5). Only once all modalities of investigations like endoscopic, radiographic, and surgical examination reveal no cause can a case be branded as idiopathic. Gacek et al.[7] explain the

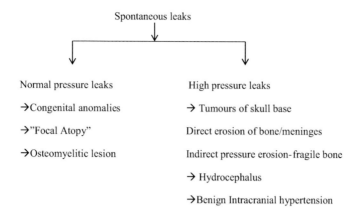

Figure 3.4 Classification of CSF leaks: spontaneous/non-traumatic leaks. © Jyotirmay S Hegde, Hemanth Vamanshankar.

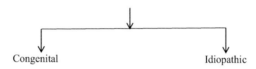

Figure 3.5 Classification of CSF leaks: congenital/idiopathic CSF rhinorrhea. © Jyotirmay S Hegde, Hemanth Vamanshankar.

probable cause of idiopathic CSF leaks based on arachnoid granulations present in the temporal bone, roofs of sphenoid and ethmoid sinuses. These granulations are not covered by endothelium and are connected directly to dural extensions. Pulsations of such granulations cause localized destruction of the underlying bone.

## TAKE-HOME POINTS

- Ommaya et al. classification is one of the oldest and is the most used.
- Classification based on site, traumatic, spontaneous, and congenital/idio-pathic are other classifications for CSF leaks.
- Good history taking is a must. Sometimes a spontaneous leak may be an old case of a traumatic leak.

## REFERENCES

1. Cairns H. Injuries of the frontal and ethmoidal sinuses with special reference to cerebrospinal fluid rhinorrhoea and aeroceles. *J Laryngol Otol* 52: 589–623, 1937.

2. O'Connell JEA. Primary spontaneous cerebrospinal fluid rhinorrhoea. *J Neurol Neurosurg Psychiatry* 27: 241–6, 1964.
3. Ommaya AK, Chiro DG, Baldwin M, Pennybackeri JB. Non-traumatic cerebrospinal fluid rhinorrhoea. *J Neurol Neurosurg Psychiatry* 31: 214–25, 1968.
4. Har-El G. What is "spontaneous" cerebrospinal fluid rhinorrhoea? Classification of cerebrospinal fluid leaks. *Ann Otol Rhinol Laryngol* 108: 323–6, 1999.
5. Crawford C, Kennedy N, Weir WR. Cerebrospinal fluid rhinorrhoea and *Hemophilus influenzae* meningitis 37 years after a head injury. *J Infect* 28: 93–7, 1994.
6. Rovit RL, Shechter MM, Nelson K. Spontaneous "high pressure cerebro-spinal rhinorrhoea" due to lesions obstructing flow of cerebrospinal fluid. *J Neurosurg* 30: 406–12, 1969.
7. Gacek RR. Arachnoid granulation cerebrospinal fluid otorrhea. *Ann Otol Rhinol Laryngol* 99: 854–62, 1990.

# 4

# Spontaneous CSF rhinorrhea

## HEMANTH VAMANSHANKAR AND JYOTIRMAY S HEGDE

St Clair Thomson, in his monograph in 1899, first attempted to describe the term "spontaneous cerebrospinal rhinorrhea". In 1964, in a classification of cerebrospinal leaks written by Ommaya et al., the term "non-traumatic leaks" was used instead of "spontaneous leaks".[1]

The word "spontaneous" means "developing without apparent external influence or force or from some undiscoverable cause".[2] It has been described as one without a history of trauma, congenital defect, or infection by Pappas et al.[3,4] May et al. refer to a spontaneous leak when there is no history of trauma or congenital defect elicited.[5]

Spontaneous or non-traumatic leaks are further subclassified into high pressure or normal pressure leaks (Figure 4.1).[1] High-pressure leaks may be due to tumors (which in turn could either cause direct erosion of the meninges and leak, or indirectly by pressure erosion of the anatomically fragile areas of the skull base, especially the cribriform plate) or hydrocephalus (both obstructive and communicating). Congenital anomalies like Crouzon's disease and Albers-Schönberg disease may also rarely be associated with hydrocephalus, thus causing high-pressure leaks. Congenital anomalies with normal pressure leaks would usually present as a nasal encephalocele. Rarely, erosion due to osteomyelitis has been described as the case of a normal pressure leak. Such an explanation was given by Nori and Carteri in 1964. "Focal atrophy" described by Ommaya et al., is a speculative cause for normal pressure leak.[1]

Spontaneous cerebrospinal leaks are rare, with an incidence ranging from 3–23%, according to various authors.[6–8] Obese, middle-aged female patients (usually in their fourth decade of life) most commonly present with this condition, with a male-to-female ratio of 1:2.[6] Patients usually present with clear watery rhinorrhea, headache, pulsatile tinnitus, and visual disturbances, and most commonly have an associated increase in intracranial pressure.[9]

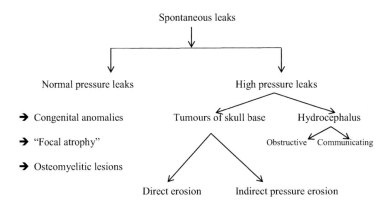

Figure 4.1 Classification of spontaneous CSF Leaks. © Jyotirmay S Hegde, Hemanth Vamanshankar.

Various theories have been put forth for the possible cause of spontaneous cerebrospinal leaks. Gacek proposed that arachnoid granulations are covered by dural extensions, since they do not extend into a venous sinus lumen. Destruction of the surrounding bone is thus seen when pulsations are transmitted through the capsule of arachnoid granulations, due to a closed system of CSF within.[10] According to Ommaya's focal atrophy theory, ischemia causes a reduction in bulk of the normal contents of cribriform plate and sella turcica. Arachnoid pouches filled with CSF tend to occupy these empty spaces; the pulsatile pressure of CSF

## THEORY OF SPONTANEOUS CSF LEAK

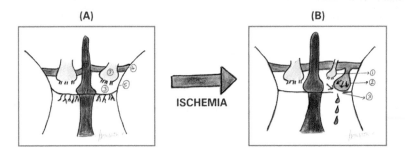

**CRIBRIFORM PLATE ANATOMY**

1. Crista Galli
2. Cranial Nerve-1
3. Cribriform Plate
4. Lateral Lamella
5. Subarachnoid Space with CSF

1. Atrophy of contents of cribriform plate due to ischemia
2. Pulsatile arachnoid granulations occupying cribriform plate area
3. Eroded cribriform plate with CSF rhinorrhoea

Figure 4.2 (A) Anatomy of the cribriform plate (B) Proposed theory of spontaneous CSF leak. © Jyotirmay S Hegde, Hemanth Vamanshankar.

creates a focal erosive effect on the underlying bone[1] (Figure 4.2 A, B). As spontaneous cerebrospinal leaks are usually associated with raised intracranial tension (benign intracranial hypertension or pseudotumor cerebri), Locke proposed that the exaggerated flow of CSF in these causes expansion and rupture of the arachnoid sleeve around olfactory filaments at the cribriform plate.[11] Intracranial pressures usually exceed 20 cm $H_2O$ in these cases.[12] In sphenoid sinus leaks, extensive pneumatisation of the sinus into the greater wings, in addition to the pterygoid process, with the presence of arachnoid villi pits in the middle cranial fossa, causes bony erosions over a period of time.[13,14]

Spontaneous leaks most commonly occur in the cribriform plate, sphenoid sinus, and anterior ethmoids; less commonly in the frontal sinus, posterior ethmoids, and inferior clivus. The cribriform plate, apart from being the site of maldevelopment, also has extension of the subarachnoid space through its foramina, thus making it particularly vulnerable to such leaks.[15]

Of special mention are the sphenoid sinus spontaneous leaks which, although rare, are more common in this location than secondary leaks. Embryologically, the sphenoid bone develops from four parts: the presphenoid (forming the anterior sphenoid bone); the basisphenoid (forming the posterior sphenoid bone); the orbitosphenoid (forming lesser wings); and the alisphenoid (forming greater wings and lateral parts of the pterygoid process). Neonatal bones have a weak cartilaginous connection between the central and lateral parts – the fusion of which occurs after birth – from the anterior to posterior regions. Just before complete fusion, a canal-connecting middle cranial fossa and nasopharynx called the "lateral craniophangeal" or Sternberg's canal (named after Sternberg in 1888, although first described by Cruveilhier in 1877) is formed (Figure 4.3). This canal closes by the age of ten years through ossification. Persistence of this canal into adulthood may be the cause

## DEVELOPMENT OF SPHENOID BONE

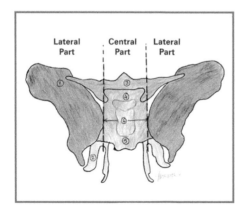

1. Alisphenoid
2. Membranous Part
3. Orbito-Sphenoid
4. Pre-Sphenoid
5. Basi Sphenoid
6. Weak cartilaginous connection between central & lateral parts of fusion ➝ persistence of which forms the Sternberg's canal.

Figure 4.3 Development of the sphenoid bone. © Jyotirmay S Hegde, Hemanth Vamanshankar.

of a potential CSF leak.[16] Possible sites of sphenoid defects include: the upper roof of the lateral recess of sphenoid sinus; persistent Sternberg's canal (incidence ranges from 0.42–6.1%); the parasellar region; and the roof of the sphenoid.[16]

Radiological investigations may give a clue to the diagnosis of spontaneous CSF leaks. High-resolution computed tomography (CT) scans may reveal attenuation and thinning of the skull base, arachnoid pits due to bony impressions from the arachnoid villi,[13] dehiscence of the ethmoid roof,[17] and pneumatisation of the lateral sphenoid recess.[18] Small ventricles, encephaloceles, a partial or complete empty sella and dilated optic nerve sheath complex may be seen on magnetic resonance imaging (MRI).[9,19]

Intrathecal sodium fluorescein, first used by Kirshner in 1960, and further developed by Messerklinger, is administered 1–2 hours prior to the surgical procedure. Its viewing is enhanced with a blue light filter intraoperatively. One of the many recommended dilution protocols that is followed is 0.1 mL of 10% sodium fluorescein in 10 mL of CSF, this mixture is used for a slow intrathecal injection for over 10 minutes; following which the patient is kept in the Trendelenburg position.[20] Topical application of 5% fluorescein intranasally, and looking for change in the color of the cotton pledget from yellow to green, is recommended by some authors.[21]

Conservative management includes reducing intracranial pressure by nursing in a semi-Fowler's position, avoiding increasing intraabdominal pressure, avoiding nose blowing, sneezing and straining, and the administration of antibiotic and carbonic anhydrase inhibitors. Conservative treatment, however, has a success rate of only 50%.[22] One should remember that in the case of a spontaneous leak, a conservative attitude is only justifiable in patients of high-pressure leaks where the causal agent cannot be removed.[1]

Endoscopic repair is now considered superior in the treatment of spontaneous CSF rhinorrhea, with a success rate varying between 76–95%.[23] However, endoscopic repair has its limits, and may not be applicable in the case of defects greater than 3 cm in diameter or defects in frontal sinus with prominent lateral extension.[6] Complications of endoscopic repair include: frontal lobe abscess, transient hemiparesis, nasal adhesions, and septal perforations, meningitis, and pneumoacephalus.[6] Failure rates after a first attempt, as compared to the CSF leak of other etiologies, is high-ranging, being from 25–87%.[6,24–28] Failures here can also cause a subsequent leak at a site other than that of repair. The main cause of failure is the lack of managing elevated intracranial pressure, which is most commonly seen in these types of leaks.[22] Supplemental procedures to augment a good surgical repair are weight reduction, recording lumbar drain pressure, use of acetazolamide, and the use of a ventriculoperitoneal shunt in severe cases of benign intracranial hypertension (if pressures are higher than 35 mm of $H_2O$).[29]

## TAKE-HOME POINTS

- Spontaneous leaks are rare, most commonly seen in the region of cribriform plate.
- The majority of spontaneous leaks are secondary to intracranial hypertension.

- Obese, middle-aged female patients are more at risk.
- Surgical management is the treatment in the majority of spontaneous leaks, supplemented with conservative measures and decreasing intracranial pressure.

## REFERENCES

1. Ommaya AK, Chiro G D, Baldwin M, Pennybacker JB. Non-traumatic cerebrospinal fluid rhinorrhoea. *J Neurol Neurosurg Psychiatry* 1968; 31:214–25.
2. Gove PB (Ed.). *Webster's Third New International Dictionary.* Springfield, MA: Merriam-Webster, 1986, p. 2204.
3. Pappas DG, Hoffman RA, Cohen NL, Pappas DG. Spontaneous temporal bone cerebrospinal fluid leak. *Am J Otol* 1992; 13:534–9.
4. Pappas DG, Pappas DG, Hoffman RA, Harris SD. Spontaneous cerebrospinal fluid leaks originating from multiple skull base defects. *Skull Base Surg* 1996; 6:227–30.
5. May JS, Mikus JL, Matthews BL, Browne JD. Spontaneous cerebrospinal fluid. *Am J Otol* 1995; 16:765–71.
6. Gendeh BS, Wormald PJ, Forer M, Goh BS, Misiran K. Endoscopic repair of spontaneous cerebro-spinal fluid rhinorrhoea: A report of 3 cases. *Med J Malaysia* 2002; 57(4):503–8.
7. Stone JA, Castillo M, Neelon B, Mukherji SK. Evaluation of CSF leaks: high resolution CT compared with contrast-enhansed CT and radionuclide cisternography. *Am J Neuroradiol* 1999; 20:706–12.
8. Lindstrom DR, Toohill RJ, Loehrl TH, Smith TL. Management of cerebrospinal fluid rhinorrhea: the Medical College of Wisconsin experience. *Laryngoscope* 2004; 114:969–74.
9. Chaaban, MR, Illing E, Riley KO, Woodworth BA. Spontaneous cerebrospinal fluid leak repair: A five-year prospective evaluation. *Laryngoscope* 2014; 124:70–5.
10. Gacek RR. Arachnoid granulation cerebrospinal fluid otorrhea. *Ann Otol Rhinol Laryngol* 1990; 99:854–62.
11. Locke CE. The spontaneous escape of cerebrospinal fluid through the nose. *Arch Neurol Psychiatry* 1926; 15:309–24.
12. Schlosser R, Bolger W. Significance of empty sella in cerebrospinal fluid leaks. *Otolaryngol Head Neck Surg* 2003; 128:32–8.
13. Shetty PG, Shroff MM, Fatterpekar GM et al. A retrospective analysis of spontaneous sphenoid sinus fistula: MR and CT findings. *Am J Neuroradiol* 2000; 21:337–42.
14. Baranano CF, Cure J, Palmer JN, Woodworth BA. Sternberg's canal: Fact or fiction? *Am J Rhinol Allergy* 2009; 23:1676–71.
15. Daele J, Goffart Y, Machiels S. Traumatic, iatrogenic, and spontaneous cerebrospinal fluid (CSF) leak: Endoscopic repair. *B-ENT* 2011; 7(17):47–60.

16. Tomaszewska M, Brożek-Mądry E, Krzeski A. Spontaneous sphenoid sinus cerebrospinal fluid leak and meningoencephalocele – Are they due to patent Sternberg's canal? Videosurg Miniinv 2015; 10(2):347–58.
17. Ohnishi T. Bony defects and dehiscences of the roof of the ethmoid cells. Rhinology 1981; 19(4):195–202.
18. Bolger WE, Butzin CA, Parsons DS. Paranasal sinus bony anatomic variations and mucosal abnormalities: CT analysis for endoscopic sinus surgery. Laryngoscope 1991; 101(1 Pt 1):56–64.
19. Fiky LE, Kotb A, Mostafa BE. A unified management for spontaneous CSF leak. Int J Otolaryngol Head Neck Surg 2015; 4:141–7.
20. Wise SK, Schlosser RJ. Evaluation of spontaneous nasal cerebrospinal fluid leaks. Curr Opin Otolaryngol Head Neck Surg 2007; 15(1):28–34.
21. Saafan ME, Ragab SM, Albirmawy OA. Topical intranasal fluorescein: the missing partner in algorithms of cerebrospinal fluid fistula detection. Laryngoscope 2006; 116(7):1158–61.
22. Stankiewicz JA. Cerebrospinal fluid fistula and endoscopic sinus surgery. Laryngoscope 1991; 101(3):250–6.
23. Mattox D, Kennedy D. Endoscopic management of cerebrospinal fluid leaks and cephaloceles. Laryngoscope 1990; 100:857–62.
24. Gendeh BS, Mazita A, Selladurai BM, Jegan T, Jeevanan J, Misiran K. Endonasal endoscopic repair of anterior skull-base fistulas: the Kuala Lumpur experience. J Laryngol Otol 2000; 119(11):866–74.
25. Zweig JL, Carrau RL, Celin SE, Schaitkin BM, Pollice PA, Snyderman CH, Kassam A, Hegazy H. Endoscopic repair of cerebrospinal fluid leaks to the sinonasal tract: predictors of success. Otolaryngol Head Neck Surg 2000; 123(3):195–201.
26. Schick B, Ibing R, Brors D, Draf W. Long-term study of endonasal dura-plasty and review in the literature. Ann Otol Rhinol Laryngol 2001; 110(2):142–7.
27. Chin GY, Rice DH. Transnasal endoscopic closure of cerebrospinal fluid leaks. Laryngoscope 2003; 113(1):136–8.
28. Meco C, Arrer E, Oberascher G. Efficacy of cerebrospinal fluid fistula repair: sensitive quality control using the beta-trace protein test. Am J Rhinol 2007; 21(6):729–36.
29. Woodworth BA, Prince A, Chiu AG, Cohen NA, Schlosser RJ, Bolger WE, Kennedy DW, Palmer JN. Spontaneous CSF leaks: A paradigm for defini-tive repair and management of intracranial hypertension. Otolaryngol Head Neck Surg 2008; 138(6):715–20.

# 5

# Traumatic CSF rhinorrhea

## HEMANTH VAMANSHANKAR AND JYOTIRMAY S HEGDE

As early as 1745, the first case of CSF rhinorrhea following a traumatic skull fracture was described in literature by Bidloo the Elder. However, it was only after the advent of radiographic techniques in 1913 that Luckett described the presence of a CSF leak through an intranasal aerocele.[1] The classification system of CSF rhinorrhea was first described by the British neurosurgeon Cairns in 1937,[2] which was further elaborately defined by Ommaya, Vrabec, and Hallberg.[3,4]

Non-surgical trauma accounts for the majority (80%) of CSF leaks, 4% are non-traumatic, and 16% are accounted from surgical procedures, although the incidences from surgical trauma are increasing in number. CSF leak in traumatic cases is evident in the first two days in the majority of cases (50%), 70% by the first week, and by the end of three months in the remainder.[5,6]

The firm adherence of the dura to the anterior skull base makes it a more common site for leaks than the middle or posterior skull base.[7] The cribriform plate, being thin and fragile, is covered only by the arachnoid layer. Small fractures here easily violate the arachnoid layer in the absence of the dura. Also, the cribriform is located in the midline, below the slight medial curve of the floor of the skull base, causing CSF to gravitate to this area.[8] Sphenoid sinus (30%), frontal sinus (30%) and cribriform/ethmoid (23%) form the most common areas of leaks. However, when endoscopic surgical trauma is considered, ethmoid/cribriform (80%), frontal sinus (8%), and sphenoid sinus (4%) are the most common sites (Figure 5.1 A, B). Sphenoid sinus is the most common site after neurosurgical trauma. Temporal bone fractures can lead to CSF otorrhea and rhinorrhea.[7] 72% of temporal bone fractures lead to CSF rhinorrhea, according to Brodie and Thompson.[9]

Various classification systems have been attempted for frontobasal trauma. Five subtypes have been described by Fain et al. (Table 5.1).[10] Sakas et al., in their

## TRAUMATIC CSF LEAKS-ETIOLOGY

(A)                                         (B)

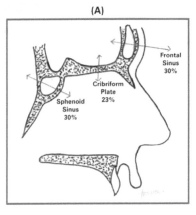
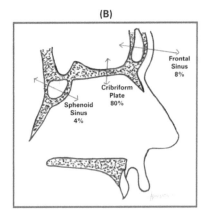

ACCIDENTAL TRAUMA                    SURGICAL TRAUMA
(BLUNT)

Figure 5.1 Etiology of traumatic CSF leaks. (A) Incidence due to accidental trauma (B) Incidence of surgical trauma. © Jyotirmay S Hegde, Hemanth Vamanshankar.

Table 5.1 Classification of frontobasal trauma by Fain et al.

| Subtype | Fain et al. – frontobasal trauma |
|---------|----------------------------------|
| Type 1 | Involvement of anterior wall of frontal sinus |
| Type 2 | Lefort Type 2 – extending upward to cranial base and anterior wall of frontal sinus |
| Type 3 | Frontal part of skull extending to cranial base |
| Type 4 | Combination of types 2 and 3 |
| Type 5 | Involvement of only sphenoid or ethmoid bones |

Table 5.2 Classification of anterior skull base fractures by Sakas et al.

| Subtype | Sakas et al. – anterior skull base fractures |
|---------|----------------------------------------------|
| Type 1 | Linear fracture through cribriform plate – without involving frontal/ethmoid sinuses |
| Type 2 | Ethmoid sinus involvement and/or medial wall of frontal sinus |
| Type 3 | Fracture through the lateral frontal sinus (superior/inferior walls) |
| Type 4 | Combination of the above |

classification, have concluded that types 1 and 2 have the highest risk of developing post-traumatic meningitis (Table 5.2).[8]

Traumatic CSF leaks present most commonly with unilateral watery rhinorrhea, which is positional and often intermittent. Acute phase (after trauma) presentations include: epistaxis, chemosis, orbital ecchymosis, anosmia, open head injury,

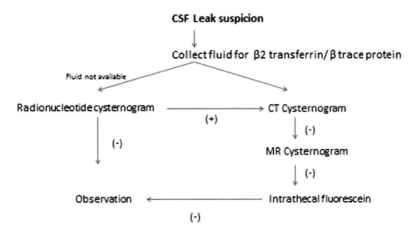

**CSF Leak suspicion**

Collect fluid for β2 transferrin/β trace protein

Fluid not available

Radionucleotide cysternogram → CT Cysternogram
(+)

(-)     (-)

MR Cysternogram

(-)

Observation ← Intrathecal fluorescein

(-)

Figure 5.2 Investigative modalities for diagnosing a CSF leak. © Jyotirmay S Hegde, Hemanth Vamanshankar.

cranial nerve deficits (most commonly the 1–3, 5 and 7th), meningitis and pneumocephalus.[11,12] Recurrent meningitis, the sensation of a sweet or salty taste in the throat, hyposmia, headaches, and intermittent nasal discharge are usually present in the chronic phase.[13,14] Paradoxical rhinorrhea (rhinorrhea from the contralateral site of the CSF leak) can result from fractures displacing midline structures, i.e., the crista galli and vomer, mucocele obstructing the ipsilateral nostril, and in temporal bone fractures. The majority of paradoxical rhinorrhea resolve spontaneously.[15,16]

Figure 5.2 below illustrates the investigative modalities of diagnosing a CSF leak in a stepwise manner.

Non-surgical/conservative management involves bed rest with head end of the bed elevation; avoiding coughing, sneezing, nose blowing; and the use of Valsalva maneuvers. 85% resolution of CSF rhinorrhea was noted by Bell et al. solely by practising conservative measures. Mincy et al. reported 68% resolution within 48 hours and 85% resolution by the first week of nonsurgical management.[17] If these measures fail, CSF diversion by means of either lumbar drain or external ventriculostomy has been advocated.[18,19] Average drainage rates are around 10 mL/hr. An overall success rate of 70–90% can be achieved when conservative management is combined with CSF diversion for an average duration of drainage of 6.5 days.[20,21]

The use of prophylactic antibiotics during this period remains controversial. The British Society of Antimicrobial Chemotherapy proposed the following arguments against the use of antibiotics. Inflamed meninges may not permit the entry of commonly used antibiotics into brain, and such treatment may lead to colonization of resistant strains; also, potential pathogens like pneumococci may not be successfully eradicated by antibiotics.[22] No significant difference in the risk of meningitis was found between groups receiving and not receiving antibiotics in CSF fistulas, according to a retrospective study by Eljamel.[23]

Conservative management can only be considered for a period of 2 weeks, failing which surgical management should be considered, as the risk of developing meningitis increases at the rate of 7.4% per week within the first month.[24] Although some authors recommend 72 hrs–7 days of bed rest followed by a 7–10-day trial of diversion maneuvers, others follow surgical management after 8 days of non-intervention failure.[8,12,25]

Surgical management is particularly required in fractures where spontaneous closures are not possible, such as a fracture with complications like tension pneumocephalus, cranial nerve deficits, a large depressed fracture, or in cases of pathologies requiring acute intervention.[11,12] Rocchi et al. suggest that surgical intervention is needed in compound, depressed, comminuted, or craniofacial fractures larger than 1 cm, fractures involving cribriform plate, or those in midline, and those injuries associated with a meningocele or encephalocele.[25]

The transcranial approach, first advocated by Dandy in 1926, by using a bifrontal craniotomy allows direct access to the defect and repair of multiple sites to be done simultaneously. However, this is fraught with morbidity from a craniotomy, and high failure rates.[24,26] In 1948, via a naso-orbital incision, Dohlman first described the extracranial approach, with a success rate of 86–97%. However, facial numbness, scarring, orbital injuries, and relative difficulty in its dissection led to it being an unfavourable approach.[27-29]

Hirsch, in 1952, reported the first transnasal approach for the repair of two sphenoid sinus CSF leaks. Other attempts to use this approach with the microscope were also carried out by Lehrer and Deutsch, but limitation of access to the superior and lateral walls of sphenoid sinus restricted such use. Also, complications like septal perforation and facial numbness were usual for this approach.[30,31]

In 1981, Wigand described the endoscopic endonasal approach. This provides best access to the cribriform plate, ethmoid roof, and sphenoid sinus. A pterygomaxillary space endoscopic dissection can be performed in leaks presenting in the lateral wall of the sphenoid sinus. Intrathecal fluorescein can be used intraoperatively for correct identification of the defect. Mucosa of about half a centimeter around the skull base defect needs to be removed prior to graft incorporation. Various autologous and non-autologous grafts have been noted in literature for their role in defect repair. These include fascia lata, temporalis fascia, mucosal grafts, muscle plugs, fat, free bone grafts (from iliac crest, septum, and calvarium), free cartilage grafts from septum or auricle, mucoperiosteal flap of the middle turbinate or a combination of these.[17] Graft placement – either onlay or inlay – yields almost similar results, according to a meta-analysis study undertaken by Hegazy et al.[32]

It is important to note that 85% of CSF leaks following head trauma resolve spontaneously. There is a 0.68% risk of developing meningitis in the first 24 hours of injury, which increases exponentially to 18.87% in the following 2 weeks after injury.[33,34] Also, a staged surgery is a preferred option: treating the intracranial pathology first, and then repair of the CSF fistula at a later stage.[11,12,26,35] Surgical intervention is a must in cases where fractures are > 1.5 cm in size, closer to the midline, if there is presence of meningoceles or encephalocele inside a fistula, and frontal sinus fractures.[11,26]

## TAKE-HOME POINTS

- The anterior skull base is more common for traumatic leaks, due to its firm adherence to the dura.
- 50% of leaks are evident by the first two days, and 70% by the first week.
- Paradoxical rhinorrhea may be one of the types of presentation.
- The majority of leaks resolve spontaneously, hence conservative management has a role. However, the risk of developing meningitis rises exponentially during this period.

## REFERENCES

1. Luckett WH. Air in the ventricle of the brain following fracture of the skull. *Surg Gynecol Obstet* 1913; 17:237–240.
2. Cairns H. Injuries of the frontal and ethmoidal sinuses with special reference to cerebrospinal fluid rhinorrhea and aeroceles. *J Laryngol Otol* 1937; 52:589–623.
3. Ommaya AK. Cerebrospinal fluid rhinorrhea. *Neurology* 1964; 14:106–113.
4. Vrabec DP, Hallberg OE. Cerebrospinal fluid rhinorrhea. Intranasal approach, review of the literature, and report of a case. *Arch Otolaryngol* 1964; 80:218–229.
5. Loew F, Pertuiset B, Chaumier EE et al. Traumatic, spontaneous and postoperative CSF rhinorrhea. *Adv Tech Stand Neurosurg* 1984; 11:169–207.
6. Kerman M, Cirak B, Dagtekin A. Management of skull base fractures. *Neurosurg Q* 2002; 12:23–41.
7. Banks CA, Palmer JN, Chiu AG et al. Endoscopic closure of CSF rhinorrhea: 193 cases over 21 years. *Otolaryngol Head Neck Surg* 2009; 140:826–33.
8. Sakas DE, Beale DJ, Ameen AA et al. Compound anterior cranial base fractures: Classification using computerized tomography scanning as a basis for selection of patients for dural repair. *J Neurosurg* 1998; 88:471–477.
9. Brodie HA, Thompson TC. Management of complications from 820 temporal bone fractures. *Am J Otol* 1997; 18:188–197.
10. Fain J, Chabannes J, Peri G et al. [Frontobasal injuries and CSF fistulas. Attempt at an anatomoclinical classification. Therapeutic incidence]. *Neurochirurgie* 1975; 21(6):493–506 [in French].
11. Scholsem M, Scholtes F, Collignon F et al. Surgical management of anterior cranial base fractures with cerebrospinal fluid fistulae: A single-institution experience. *Neurosurgery* 2008; 62:463–471.
12. Yilmazlar S, Arslan E, Kocaeli H et al. Cerebrospinal fluid leakage complicating skull base fractures: Analysis of 81 cases. *Neurosurg Rev* 2006; 29:64–71.

13. Kerr JT, Chu FW, Bayles SW. Cerebrospinal fluid rhinorrhea: Diagnosis and management. *Otolaryngol Clin North Am* 2005; 38: 597–611.
14. Cassano M, Felippu A. Endoscopic treatment of cerebrospinal fluid leaks with the use of lower turbinate grafts: A retrospective review of 125 cases. *Rhinology* 2009; 47:362–368.
15. Bhalodiya NH, Joseph ST. Cerebrospinal fluid rhinorrhea: Endoscopic repair based on a combined diagnostic approach. *Indian J Otolaryngol Head Neck Surg* 2009; 61:120–126.
16. Dalgiç A, Seçer M, Ergüngör MF et al. [Traumatic posterior fossa epidural hematomas and their complications.] *J Neurol Sci* 2007; 24:280–286 (in Turkish).
17. Mateo Z, Jennifer GS, David FJ. Diagnosis and treatment of cerebrospinal fluid rhinorrhea following accidental traumatic anterior skull base fractures. *Neurosurg Focus* 2012; 32 (6):E3.
18. Schlosser RJ, Bolger WE. Significance of empty sella in cerebrospinal fluid leaks. *Otolaryngol Head Neck Surg* 2003; 128:32–8.
19. Ratilal BO, Costa J, Sampaio C. Antibiotic prophylaxis for preventing meningitis in patients with basilar skull fractures. *Cochrane Database Syst Rev* 2006; (1):CD004884.
20. Bell RB, Dierks EJ, Homer L et al. Management of cerebrospinal fluid leak associated with craniomaxillofacial trauma. *J Oral Maxillofac Surg* 2004; 62(6):676–84.
21. Shapiro SA, Scully T. Closed continuous drainage of cerebrospinal fluid via a lumbar subarachnoid catheter for treatment of prevention of cranial/spinal cerebrospinal fluid fistula. *Neurosurgery* 1992; 30(2):241–5.
22. Anonymous. Management of cerebrospinal fluid leaks. *J Trauma* 2001; 51 (2 Suppl):S29–S33.
23. Eljamel MS. Antibiotic prophylaxis in unrepaired CSF fistulae. *Br J Neurosurg* 1993; 7:501–505.
24. Dandy WE. Treatment of rhinorrhea and otorrhea. *Arch Surg* 1944; 49:75–85.
25. Rocchi G, Caroli E, Belli E et al. Severe craniofacial fractures with frontobasal involvement and cerebrospinal fluid fistula: Indications for surgical repair. *Surg Neurol* 2005; 63:559–564.
26. Ray BS, Bergland RM. Cerebrospinal fluid fistula: Clinical aspects, techniques of localization and methods of closure. *J Neurosurg* 1967; 30:399–405.
27. Dohlman G. Spontaneous cerebrospinal fluid rhinorrhea. *Acta Otolaryngol Suppl (Stockh)* 1948; 67:20–3.
28. McCormack B, Cooper PR, Persky M et al. Extracranial repair of cerebrospinalfluid fistulas: Technique and results in 37 patients. *Neurosurgery* 1990; 27:412–7.
29. Persky MS, Rothstein SG, Breda SD et al. Extracranial repair of cerebrospinal fluid otorhinorrhea. *Laryngoscope* 1991; 101:134–6.

30. Hirsch O. Successful closure of cerebrospinal fluid rhinorrhea by endonasal surgery. *Arch Otolaryngol* 1952; 56:1–13.
31. Lehrer J, Deutsch H. Intranasal surgery for cerebrospinal fluid rhinorrhea. *Mt Sinai J Med* 1970; 37:113–38.
32. Hegazy HM, Carrau RL, Snyderman CH, Kassam A, Zweig J. Transnasal endoscopic repair of cerebrospinal fluid rhinorrhea: A meta-analysis. *Laryngoscope* 2000; 110:1166–1172.
33. Eljamel MS, Foy PM. Acute traumatic CSF fistulae: The risk of intracranial infection. *Br J Neurosurg* 1990; 4:381–385.
34. Mincy JE. Posttraumatic cerebrospinal fluid fistula of the frontal fossa. *J Trauma* 1966; 6:618–622.
35. Friedman JA, Ebersold MJ, Quast LM. Post-traumatic cerebrospinal fluid leakage. *World J Surg* 2001; 25:1062–1066.

# 6

# Iatrogenic CSF rhinorrhea

## HEMANTH VAMANSHANKAR AND JYOTIRMAY S HEGDE

Complications of the skull base and intranasal surgery in the early 20th century was so dreaded that it prompted Dr Mosher to say "surgery in this region should be simple, but it has proven to be one of the easiest ways to kill a patient" with regards to an intranasal ethmoidectomy.[1] Nonetheless, over the years, with the advent of the endoscope the surgery has become simpler and more accessible. However, it demands skill and has a learning curve. In his study, Dr Stankiewicz clearly shows how endoscopic surgery complications reduce with improved experience. His early experience using the endoscope had an overall complication rate of 29%, with major complications amounting to 8%. Over the years, with increased experience and better techniques, the major complications were reduced to 2%.[2]

## CLASSIFICATION

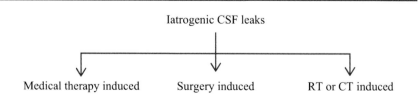

# MEDICAL THERAPY-INDUCED CSF LEAKS

CSF rhinorrhea following medical treatment for invasive tumors of the pituitary is uncommon. It is mostly seen in the setting of an invasive macroprolactinoma. Prolactinomas are the most common pituitary adenomas. Gene mutations in MEN 1 (multiple endocrine neoplasia) and aryl hydrocarbon interacting protein gene (AIP) are seen in familial types. Macroprolactinomas are defined as those which are more than 1 cm in size, while giant macroprolactinomas are those which are > 4 cm in size.[3-6] Macroprolactinomas are more common in men, and the diagnosis in them may be delayed. They account for 0.5–4.4% of pituitary tumors. Invasiveness of the prolactinomas is due to excessive secretion of matrix metalloproteinase 9, reduction of e-cadherin expression and up-regulation of protease-activated receptor 1 (PAR1).[7-9]

Dopaminergic agonists (DA) are considered to be first-line therapy in invasive macroadenomas and effectively cause tumor shrinkage. Bromocriptine, and more recently cabergoline, are used as mainstay treatment options. However, cabergoline is more effective due to higher pituitary tumor shrinkage, higher efficiency of normalizing prolactin levels, and superior affinity for dopamine receptor binding.[10-13]

CSF rhinorrhea in this setting can occur as a complication of starting DAs for tumor shrinkage (6.1% incidence), or rarely as a spontaneous leak in such invasive tumors (2.6% incidence).[14] The mechanism of a CSF leak as a complication of starting DA therapy is that the invasive tumor has the propensity to invade dura and bone. Hence, a CSF fistula is formed when the arachnoid and/or the brain parenchyma is violated. The tumor, however, occludes such a fistula like a plug. DA therapy induces rapid shrinkage of the tumor, thus facilitating a leak (Figure 6.1). Spontaneous rhinorrhea in these tumors could be related to hemorrhage and/or intratumoral infarction-induced shrinkage.[15,16]

In a review article, Lam et al. described CSF leaks in 52 patients in studies done from 1980–2011. Of these, 73% of leaks occurred following medical therapy and 27% occurred spontaneously. The mean age of occurrence was 42.8 years. 35 of the patients were males and prolactinomas accounted for 82% of the tumors. Other tumors causing leak were ACTH-secreting adenomas, GH-secreting adenomas, and nonfunctioning adenomas. The average time of developing a CSF rhinorrhea after therapy initiation was 3.3 months. Interestingly, the average initial prolactin level in those patients with medically induced leaks was 4917 ng/ml, as compared to 9169 ng/ml in patients with spontaneous onset leaks.[17]

Discontinuation of the DA agent has been shown to cause cessation of a CSF leak, possibly due to tumor re-expansion.[18] However, this may not prevent the patient from developing meningitis and pneumocephalus, and thus an eventual surgical repair is a must in these patients.[17] De Lacy et al. recommend continuation of such DA therapy even in the setting of a CSF leak, in order to prevent a tumor recurrence.[19] In patients who are not surgically fit, a conservative approach with medical therapy cessation and temporary insertion of a lumbar drain may be recommended.[17] Patients having a high flow leak may further need an external

## MECHANISM OF CSF LEAK FOLLOWING MEDICAL THERAPY IN SKULL BASE TUMORS

(A)

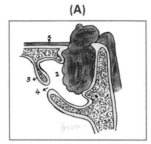

(B)

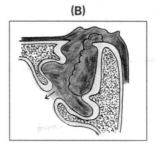

1. Tumor
2. Sphenoid Sinus
3. Anterior Wall Of Sinus
4. Sinus Opening
5. Subarachnoid Space With CSF

**Tumor Shrinkage Causing CSF Leak
(Following Medical Therapy with
eg. Dopaminergic Agonists)**

Figure 6.1 Mechanism of CSF leak following medical therapy to skull base tumors. (Reproduced by permission from Ref 42). (A) Tumor prior to medical therapy and (B) Tumor after medical therapy causing a CSF leakage. © Jyotirmay S Hegde, Hemanth Vamanshankar.

lumbar drain; those with underlying intracranial hypertension may require a permanent lumboperitoneal or ventriculoperitoneal shunt procedure.[18]

## CT- AND RT-INDUCED CSF RHINORRHEA

Yamada et al. described a case of a CyberKnife therapy-induced CSF leak for the treatment of skull base osteosarcoma. A patient presented one month after radiation with signs of meningitis and CSF leak. Although considered safer than conventional gamma knife therapy in the preservation of optic nerve function, the cause of the CSF leak was postulated to be due to dural shrinkage in a preexisting iatrogenic dural defect.[20] Kim et al. describe another case of a spontaneous CSF leak in a patient, four months after completing gamma knife surgery for metastatic renal cell carcinoma to the skull base.[21] Gamma knife-induced CSF leakage for the treatment of skull base tumors has also been described.[21-23]

Erlotinib-induced CSF rhinorrhea has been noted in a case of EGFR mutant stage 4 adenocarcinoma lung with clival and sellar metastasis, approximately one month after initiating chemotherapy.[24] A similar report following sunitinib chemotherapy for a case of recurrent atypical meningioma has been described.[25]Again, the cause of leak in these cases would probably be the shrinkage of the tumor in the aftermath of a fistula formation by the neoplastic process.[24]

Panda et al. describe a case of flutamide induced-CSF rhinorrhea while treating a Radkowski stage 3B juvenile nasopharyngeal angiofibroma (JNA). This benign locally invasive tumor is not known to invade dura or cause bony erosion.

The authors have suggested that there could be a reduction of bone mineral density precipitating a leak through an already thinned out skull base. Also, the spread of the tumor into the anterior cranial fossa through dural sleeves along the olfactory fibers, roof of the posterior ethmoid and sphenoid sinus, which is not a routine finding in the case of JNA could have also caused the leak.[26]

## SURGICALLY INDUCED CSF LEAKS

The most common sites of CSF leak following endoscopic sinus surgery are: cribriform plate and ethmoid (80%), frontal sinus (8%), and sphenoid sinus (4%).[27] In the cribriform region, iatrogenic leaks are most common in the lateral wall of the olfactory fossa and fovea ethmoidalis, which is also the medial limit of the frontal recess region. The bone at this region is very thin, ranging from 0.1–1 mm, and is usually damaged if surgical instruments are turned medially during surgery in this region. Also present in this region is the anterior ethmoidal artery. An attempt to use diathermy (especially unipolar) here in order to obtain hemostasis may burn through the bone and dura, thus causing a CSF fistula.[28] Attempts to remove cells present on the skull base near the fovea ethmoidalis could be a cause of the leak.[29]

In their study assessing the risk factors for developing CSF leaks in endonasal surgery, Ivan et al. opine that an abnormal BMI significantly predicted an increased risk for a post-operative CSF leak and meningitis. Factors like prior history of surgery, chemotherapy, radiation, tumor pathology or location, pre-op lumbar drain insertion were not associated with an increased risk of CSF leak.[29]

Rates of CSF rhinorrhea after endonasal surgeries vary from 15–25%. However, with the use of vascular flaps instead of mucosal free grafts, these rates have dropped to < 6%.[30–32] Further, the size of the dural defect, the extent of the intraoperative CSF leak, whether the leak is a high flow or low flow, surgical entry into the ventricle, correct positioning, counter-pressure of the nasoseptal flap, and surgical training and expertise contribute to the viability of a nasoseptal flap.[29] Post-operative CSF leak is also more common in obese, middle-aged females with idiopathic increased intracranial pressure.[33]

Abobotain et al. reported a case of CSF rhinorrhea following submucosal diathermy of the inferior turbinate three weeks after the said surgery. The fistula was located in the nasopharynx at the craniocervical junction. The diathermy probe which is 10 cm in size had pierced through the nasopharynx, just short of the basilar artery[34] (which is usually at a distance of 110–130 mm, with a mean of 110 mm from the anterior choana[35]). Also, in nasal surgery, the incidence of complications is more in right-sided surgery as compared to the left side – as observed in the above case.[36]

Seven cases of iatrogenic post-septoplasty-induced CSF leak with defects in the cribriform plate have been reported in literature.[37]

Adenoidectomy-induced CSF leaks have been reported. Two cases were seen in the conventional approach of adenoidectomy: one due to extensive cautery use to control bleeding, and the other due to excessive curettage and injuring the medial pterygopalatine fossa in a child with a congenital bony defect.[38,39] Morena et al. reported a case of a trans-oral endoscopic approach-associated adenoid-ectomy causing a CSF leak and pneumocephalus. Ramasamy et al. noted a case of CSF rhinorrhea with pneumocephalus, secondary to the use of the microde-brider in adenoidectomy. They postulated that overzealous removal associated with a marked diminution of tactile feedback may have caused the damage at the cranio-cervical junction in the nasopharynx.[40]

A case of CSF rhinorrhea from the ethmoid roof following balloon dilatation in a revision sinus surgery was reported by Sayal et al.[41]

## TAKE-HOME POINTS

- Iatrogenic leaks may be classified into medical therapy-induced, surgical-therapy induced and chemotherapy- or radiotherapy-induced.
- Medical therapy induced-CSF leak is mainly seen in the setting of dopaminergic agonist-induced shrinkage of invasive macroprolactinomas.
- The most common sites of surgically induced leaks are seen in cribriform and ethmoid region, frontal sinus, and sphenoid sinuses.
- Incidence rates of surgical leaks vary from 15-25%.

## REFERENCES

1. Mosher HP (1929) The symposium of the ethmoid-a surgical anatomy of the ethmoidal labyrinth. In *Trans 34th Ann Meet Am Acad Ophthamology and Otolaryngology*. vol. 34, pp. 376–410.
2. Stankiewicz JA (1987) Complications of endoscopic intranasal ethmoidec-tomy. *Laryngoscope* 97:1270–1273.
3. Wong A, Eloy JA, Couldwell WT, Liu JK (2015) Update on prolactinomas. Part 1: Clinical manifestations and diagnostic challenges. *J Clin Neurosci* 22(10):1562–1567.
4. Schlechte JA (2003) Clinical practice. Prolactinoma. *N Engl J Med* 349(21):2035–2041.
5. Mindermann T, Wilson CB (1994) Age-related and gender related occur-rence of pituitary adenomas. *Clin Endocrinol* 41(3):359–364.
6. Beckers A, Daly AF (2007) The clinical, pathological, and genetic features of familial isolated pituitary adenomas. *Eur J Endocrinol* 157(4):371–382.
7. Giraudo E, Inoue M, Hanahan D (2004) An amino-bisphosphonate targets MMP-9-expressing macrophages and angiogenesis to impair cervical carcinogenesis. *J Clin Invest* 114(5):623–633.
8. Qian ZR, Li CC, Yamasaki H et al. (2002) Role of E-cadherin, α-, β-, and γ-catenins, and p120 (cell adhesion molecules) in prolactinoma behavior. *Mod Pathol* 15(12):1357–1365.
9. Darmoul D, Gratio V, Devaud H et al. (2003) Aberrant expression and activation of the thrombin receptor protease-activated receptor-1 induces cell proliferation and motility in human colon cancer cells. *Am J Pathol* 162(5):1503–1513.

10. Melmed S, Casanueva FF, Hoffman AR et al. (2011) Endocrine Society. Diagnosis and treatment of hyperprolactinemia: An Endocrine Society clinical practice guideline. *J Clin Endocrinol Metab* 96(2):273–288.

11. Knoepfelmacher M, Gomes MC, Melo ME, Mendonca BB (2004) Pituitary apoplexy during therapy with cabergoline in an adolescent male with prolactin-secreting macroadenoma. *Pituitary* 7(2):83–87.

12. Wong A, Eloy JA, Couldwell WT, Liu JK (2015) Update on prolactinomas. Part 2: Treatment and management strategies. *J Clin Neurosci* 22(10):1568–1574.

13. Verhelst J, Abs R, Maiter D et al. (1999) Cabergoline in the treatment of hyperprolactinemia: A study in 455 patients. *J Clin Endocrinol Metab* 84(7):2518–2522.

14. Suliman SG, Gurlek A, Byrne JV et al. (2007) Nonsurgical cerebrospinal fluid rhinorrhea in invasive macroprolactinoma: Incidence, radiological, and clinicopathological features. *J Clin Endocrinol Metab* 92:3829–3835. doi: 10.1210/jc.2007-0373

15. Kok JG, Bartelink AK, Schulte BP et al. (1985) Cerebrospinal fluid rhinorrhea during treatment with bromocriptine for prolactinoma. *Neurology* 35:1193–1195.

16. Landolt AM (1982) Cerebrospinal fluid rhinorrhea: A complication of therapy for invasive prolactinomas. *Neurosurgery* 11:395–401.

17. Lam G, Mehta V, Zada G (2012) Spontaneous and medically induced cerebrospinal fluid leakage in the setting of pituitary adenomas: Review of the literature. *Neurosurg Focus* 32(6):E2.

18. Česák T, Poczos P, Adamkov J et al. (2018) Medically induced CSF rhinorrhea following treatment of macroprolactinoma: Case series and literature review. *Pituitary* 21(6):561–570. doi: 10.1007/s11102-018-0907-1

19. De Lacy P, Benjamin S, Dixon R et al. (2009) Is surgical intervention frequently required for medically managed macroprolactinomas? A study of spontaneous cerebrospinal fluid rhinorrhea. *Surg Neurol* 72(5):461–463.

20. Yamada SM, Ishii Y, Yamada S et al. (2013) Skull base osteosarcoma presenting with cerebrospinal fluid leakage after CyberKnife treatment: A case report. *J Med Case Rep* 7:116.

21. Kim CH, Chung SK, Dhong HJ, Lee JI (2008) Cerebrospinal fluid leakage after gamma knife radiosurgery for skull base metastasis from renal cell carcinoma: A case report. *Laryngoscope* 118:1925–1927.

22. Ogawa Y, Tominaga T (2007) Delayed cerebrospinal fluid leakage 10 years after transsphenoidal surgery and gamma knife surgery – Case report. *Neurol Med Chir* 47:483–485.

23. Hongmei Y, Zhe W, Jing W et al. (2012) Delayed cerebrospinal fluid rhinorrhea after gamma knife surgery in a patient with a growth hormone-secreting adenoma. *J Clin Neurosci* 19:900–902.

24. Priddy B, Hardesty DA, Beer-Furlan A et al. (2017) Cerebrospinal fluid leak rhinorrhea after systemic erlotinib chemotherapy for metastatic lung cancer: A familiar problem from an unfamiliar culprit. *Case Rep* 108:992. e11–992.e14. doi: 10.1016/j.wneu.2017.08.183

25. Raheja A, Colman H, Palmer CA, Couldwell WT (2016) Dramatic radiographic response resulting in cerebrospinal fluid rhinorrhea associated with sunitinib therapy in recurrent atypical meningioma: Case report. *J Neurosurg* 9:1–6.

26. Panda S, Phalak M, Thakar A, Krishnan S (2018) CSF Leak in juvenile nasopharyngeal angiofibroma – Rare sequelae of flutamide induced tumour shrinkage. *World Neurosurg* 120:78–81. doi: 10.1016/j.wneu.2018.07.288

27. Prosser DJ, Vender JR, Solares CA (2011) Traumatic cerebrospinal fluid leaks. *Otolaryngol Clin N Am* 44:857–873.

28. Wormald PJ (2008) *Endoscopic Sinus Surgery. Anatomy, Three Dimensional Reconstruction, and Surgical Technique* (2nd edition). New York: Thieme.

29. Ivan ME, Iorgulescu JB, El-Sayed I et al. (2015) Risk factors for postoperative cerebrospinal fluid leak and meningitis after expanded endoscopic endonasal surgery. *J Clin Neurosci* 22:48–54.

30. de Divitiis E, Cavallo LM, Esposito F et al. (2007) Extended endoscopic transsphenoidal approach for tuberculum sellae meningiomas. *Neurosurgery* 61:229–37 [discussion 237–8].

31. Stamm AC, Vellutini E, Harvey RJ et al. (2008) Endoscopic transnasal craniotomy and the resection of craniopharyngioma. *Laryngoscope* 118:1142–1148.

32. Kassam AB, Prevedello DM, Carrau RL et al. (2011) Endoscopic endonasal skull base surgery: Analysis of complications in the authors' initial 800 patients. *J Neurosurg* 114:1544–1568.

33. Snyderman CH, Kassam AB, Carrau R et al. (2007) Endoscopic reconstruction of cranial base defects following endonasal skull base surgery. *Skull Base* 17:73–78.

34. Abobotain AH, Ajlan A, Alsaleh S (2018) Cerebrospinal fluid leakage after turbinate submucosal diathermy: An unusual complication. *Ann Saudi Med* 38:143–147.

35. Lai LT, Morgan MK, Chin DC et al. (2013) A cadaveric study of the endoscopic endonasal transclival approach to the basilar artery. *J Clin Neurosci* 20(4):587–592. doi: 10.1016/j. jocn.2012.03.042

36. Hosemann W, Draf C (2013) Danger points, complications and medico-legal aspects in endoscopic sinus surgery. *GMS Curr Top Otorhinolaryngol Head Neck Surg* 12:Doc06.1. doi: 10.3205/cto000098

37. Venkatesan N, Mattox DE, Del Gaudio JM (2014) Cerebrospinal fluid leaks following septoplasty. *Ear Nose Throat J* 93:43–46.

38. Benítez L, Fernández A, Sánchez C (2013) Cerebrospinal fluid leak after adenoidectomy: A case report. *Eur J Anaesthesiol* 30:157.

39. Vassos G, Kong J, Hopkins C et al. (2012) Case report: CSF leak developed after adenoidectomy. *J Neurol Surg B*, 73:A460.
40. Ramasamy K, Vamanshankar H, Saxena SK et al. (2018) Cranio-cervical junction cerebrospinal fluid leak after microdebrider-assisted adenoidectomy – A rare case report. *Acta Otorrinolaringol Esp* 69:53–55. doi: 10.1016/j.otorri.2017.01.006
41. Sayal NR, Keider E, Korkigian S (2018) Visualized ethmoid roof cerebrospinal fluid leak during frontal balloon sinuplasty. *Ear Nose Throat J* 97(8):E34–E38.
42. Kalinin PL, Shkarubo AN, Astafieva LI et al. Cerebrospinal fluid rhinorrhea in primary treatment of large and giant prolactinomas with dopamine agonists. *Voprosy neĭrokhirurgii* 81:32. doi: 10.17116/neiro201781632-39

# 7

# Idiopathic intracranial hypertension and CSF rhinorrhea

HEMANTH VAMANSHANKAR AND JYOTIRMAY S HEGDE

Idiopathic intracranial hypertension (IIH) may be defined as a syndrome comprising of CSF having a normal fluid composition presenting with symptoms of raised intracranial pressure, in the absence of a mass lesion or ventriculomegaly.[1] Although initially named as benign intracranial hypertension and pseudotumor cerebri, these terms are no longer accepted as the condition causes significant visual morbidity, and the term "pseudotumor" gives a false impression that the disease is not real.[2] IIH has an estimated incidence of 0.9 per 100,000 population – but this increases to 20 per 100,000 in obese childbearing women.[3]

The modified Dandy's criteria for a diagnosis of IIH (2002) are as follows:[3]

1. Signs and symptoms of papilledema or generalized intracranial hypertension.
2. Elevated intracranial pressures documented in the lateral decubitus position.
3. Normal CSF composition.
4. No evidence of hydrocephalus, mass, structural, or vascular lesion seen on computed tomography (CT) or magnetic resonance imaging (MRI).
5. No identified cause of intracranial hypertension.

The fact that IIH is often seen as a cause for a spontaneous CSF leak has led to a few authors suggesting that primary spontaneous leaks may represent a form of IIH.[4–10]

The exact etiology of IIH is not known, although a lot of theories have been proposed. The roles of adipose tissue behaving as an actively secreting endocrine tissue, vitamin A metabolism, and central venous abnormalities have been researched. Obstruction of CSF drainage at the arachnoid villi, which is seen in 84% of patients of IIH, is probably the most accepted theory. Farb et al. proposed that chronically elevated ICP causes remodeling of the skull base and rupture of the arachnoid sleeve surrounding olfactory filaments in the cribriform plate region, thus causing a CSF leak.[11] In the case of sphenoid leaks, the empty sella seen in these conditions may allow transmission of increased CSF pulsation through an incompetent diaphragm sellae, which in due course causes sellar erosion and CSF leak.[12,13]

Obesity is seen as an independent risk factor for spontaneous development of CSF leaks. Visceral obesity causes increased intra-abdominal pressure, which in turn causes an increase in central venous pressure. According to Dlouhy et al., an obesity-induced increase in pleural and cardiac filling pressures may decrease venous return from the brain, thus contributing to a raised ICP seen in IIH. Also, obesity causes elevation in the levels of coagulation factors, lipoprotein (a), and plasminogen activator inhibitor-1, which in turn cause endothelial dysfunction and platelet aggregation abnormality. This can contribute to the development of occult thrombosis of dural venous sinuses and microthrombi in arachnoid granulations.[14] In a retrospective study of 4235 patients it was observed that a unit increase in BMI caused a 0.24 mmHg increase in ICP.[15]

Obstructive sleep apnoea (OSA) is also known to be commonly associated with IIH. An intermittent elevation of ICP during episodes of apnoea and persistent raised ICP during awake states is seen in OSA patients. Spontaneous CSF rhinorrhea patients had a 2.85–4.73% more likelihood to have OSA in a meta-analytical study.[16]

The most common sites of leak are the lateral wall of the sphenoid sinus and ethmoid.[5]

Although signs/symptoms of raised ICT (headache, tinnitus, visual disturbances, and neck stiffness) can occur in active leaks, in the majority of instances the clinical features of raised intracranial hypertension manifest only after the CSF leak has been closed. Sometimes, patients presenting with frank bacterial meningitis may lead to the discovery of a CSF leak.[17] Recent studies have shown that almost 94.3% patients of IIH may develop papilledema. Further, around 10–25% patients developing papilledema may develop a permanent visual loss despite therapy for the same.[18,19] A recent weight gain, subretinal hemorrhage, high grade or atrophic papilledema, significant visual field loss at presentation, and presence of hypertension are predictors of visual loss in patients with IIH.[2]

A CSF opening pressure greater than 25 cm $H_2O$ is consistent with the diagnosis of IIH.[20] The mean CSF opening pressures vary between 25–32.5 cm $H_2O$ post-repair of CSF leaks, in the absence of addressing the underlying IIH.[21]

Radiologic studies have shown that 100% of patients with spontaneous leaks with IIH have a completely or partially empty sella, compared to 5–6% in the general population and 11% in non-spontaneous leaks.[22] Tortuous optic nerves, presence of arachnoid pits, increased CSF around the optic nerves, transverse venous sinus stenosis, and dural ectasia are other findings observed on MRI.[23] CT scans may show evidence of skull base defects and enlarged foramen ovale,[24,25] thin skull base in the region of the lateral lamella, roof of the ethmoid sinus, and sella turcica.[26] CSF leaks in IIH are found to be more common over areas of increased sinus pneumatization. Conversely, patients of IIH not having significant sinus pneumatization develop ocular signs like papilledema.[25,27]

Not all patients of IIH may require treatment. It is self-limiting in some cases. Two main reasons for treating IIH (apart from CSF rhinorrhea) are optic neuropathy and intractable headache.[28] Protocol for the management of IIH is provided in Figure 7.1.

Weight loss and dietary management is of primordial importance in these patients. A low-calorie rice diet (400–1000 calorie/day) was proven to cause the rapid resolution of papilledema in nine obese patients.[29] A low-tyramine diet with a limitation of vitamin A consumption is said to be of benefit.[30,31] Carbonic anhydrase inhibitors like acetazolamide, which act by decreasing the secretion of CSF from the choroid plexus, are accepted as first-line treatment in lowering ICP. Diuretics like furosemide, spironolactone, and triamterene have also been used. Corticosteroids may be used in the short term for the rapid decrease of ICP as an adjunct surgical management.

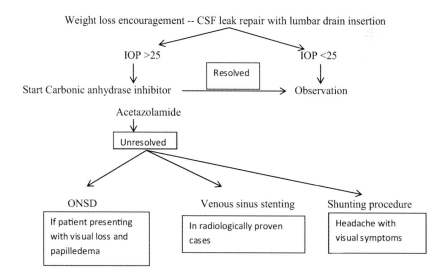

Figure 7.1 Protocol for IIH management. © Jyotirmay S Hegde, Hemanth Vamanshankar.

Treatment of systemic disorders which are known to increase ICP like hyperthyroidism, hypoparathyroidism, iron deficiency anemia, Addison's disease, sarcoidosis, and hypervitaminosis-A should be dealt with.[32] Long-term medications that are associated with increased ICP include: danazol, levodopa, carbidopa, lithium, phenytoin, oral contraceptive pills, vitamin A, and cyclosporine.[33] Hence, a multispecialty combined management may be needed in such a setting.

Lumbar punctures may be used in patients with occasional relapses, pregnancy or in cases of rapidly declining vision, prior to planning more aggressive treatment.[34] The perioperative use of lumbar drain (LD) may be indicated in the following cases:

1. In localizing difficult leaks/concurrent skull base defects by introducing intrathecal fluorescein through the LD.
2. Post-operative ICP measurement.
3. Immediate post-operative period to aid in surgical success.

## SURGICAL MANAGEMENT

1. CSF diversion procedure: Of the two modalities, lumboperitoneal shunt is preferred to ventriculoperitoneal shunt as insertion and patency maintenance is easier in the former. Shunting procedure is usually indicated in patients with ICP's > 35 cm $H_2O$, inadequate response to medical therapy with acetazolamide, and those with multiple defects.[35] However, shunt failures are known to occur, with an incidence ranging from 38–64%. The causes may include: catheter migration, infection, shunt valve migration, and cerebellar tonsil herniation.
2. Bariatric surgery: Performed in morbidly obese individuals, it reduces cardiovascular risk, lumbar disc degeneration, and type 2 diabetes mellitus.[2]
3. Optic nerve sheath decompression (ONSD): Usually carried out for refractory cases involving visual loss or intractable headaches. The possible mechanisms of benefit in IIH are overall decreasing ICP, improving peripapillary circulation, and causing a scarring effect of arachnoid over the optic nerve head, thus protecting it against an elevated CSF pressure. ONSD thus avoids the need for shunting and its complications, needs shorter anesthesia and hospitalization.[36-38]
4. Venous sinus stenting (VSS) in patients with imaging evidence of transverse sinus stenosis (secondary to septal bands, enlarged arachnoid granulations, intrinsic vessel narrowing, or extrinsic compression),[39] has been demonstrated as an effective alternate treatment modality for patients with IIH. VSS has been shown to improve clinical symptoms associated with IIH by quantitatively reducing post-procedure ICP and venous sinus pressure gradient.[40-49] Improvement in papilledema (97%), visual acuity (78%), and headaches (83%) were noted after transverse VSS in a meta-analytical study of 136 patients by Satti et al.[50]

The repair of a skull base defect is surgically challenging, as the bone fractures easily, and is attenuated. Hence, caution should be excised while undertaking a placement of the bone grafts.[51]

The rate of recurrence after surgery for spontaneous leaks (without ICP control) ranges from 25–87%. However, after adequate control of ICP, surgical success rates are about 95%.[17]

Malignant IIH is a variant of IIH presenting with rapidly progressive visual loss and papilledema. Prompt treatment with lumbar drain insertion, corticosteroids, and acetazolamide may be required prior to ONSD or a shunting procedure. IIH during pregnancy may be dealt with by serial lumbar punctures and headache management. Chlorthalidone may be preferred over acetazolamide. Surgery may be needed in rare circumstances, wherein an ONSD is preferred over shunting.[2]

The association of IIH with spontaneous leaks has been known for long. Obesity is an associated risk factor. A weight loss program, combined with a definitive protocol for management with a multidisciplinary approach is required. Early management strategies with close follow-up to prevent the development of CSF leaks and visual loss should be ensured.

## TAKE-HOME POINTS

- IIH is defined by the modified Dandy's criteria.
- Obesity is an independent risk factor for spontaneous CSF leaks, and obstructive sleep apnoea is associated with IIH.
- Most symptoms of raised ICP manifest after the CSF leak is repaired.
- Weight loss, acetazolamide, and diuretics are the first line of therapy.
- Surgical modalities of treatment include lumbar punctures, CSF diversion, bariatric surgery, optic nerve sheath decompression, and venous sinus stenting.

## REFERENCES

1. Bandyopadhyay S. Pseudotumor cerebri. *Arch Neurol* 2001; 58: 1699–701.
2. Friedman DI, Jacobson DM. Idiopathic intracranial hypertension. *J Neuro-Ophthalmol* 2004; 24(2): 138–145.
3. Durcan FJ, Corbett JJ, Wall M. The incidence of pseudotumor cerebri. Population studies in Iowa and Louisiana. *Arch Neurol* 1988; 45: 875–877.
4. Clark D, Bullock P, Hui T, et al. Benign intracranial hypertension: A cause of CSF rhinorrhoea. *J Neurol Neurosurg Psychiatry* 1994; 57: 847–849.
5. Yang Z, Wang B, Wang C, et al. Primary spontaneous cerebrospinal fluid rhinorrhea: A symptom of idiopathic intracranial hypertension? *J Neurosurg* 2011; 115: 165–170.
6. Schlosser RJ, Wilensky EM, Grady MS, et al. Elevated intracranial pressures in spontaneous cerebrospinal fluid leaks. *Am J Rhinol* 2003; 17: 191–195.

7. Schlosser RJ, Woodworth BA, Wilensky EM, et al. Spontaneous cerebrospinal fluid leaks: A variant of benign intracranial hypertension. *Ann Otol Rhinol Laryngol* 2006; 115: 495–500.

8. Suryadevara AC, Fattal M, Woods CI. Nontraumatic cerebrospinal fluid rhinorrhea as a result of pseudotumor cerebri. *Am J Otol* 2007; 28: 242–246.

9. Brainard L, Chen DA, Aziz KM, et al. Association of benign intracranial hypertension and spontaneous encephalocele with cerebrospinal fluid leak. *Otol & Neurotol* 2012; 33: 1621–1624.

10. Rudnick E, Sismanis A. Pulsatile tinnitus and spontaneous cerebrospinal fluid rhinorrhea: Indicators of benign intracranial hypertension syndrome. *Otol & Neurotol* 2005; 26: 166–168.

11. Farb RI, Vanek I, Scott JN, et al. Idiopathic intracranial hypertension. The prevalence and morphology of sinovenous stenosis. *Neurology* 2003; 60: 1418–1424.

12. Bjerre P, Lindholm J, Glydensted C. Pathogenesis of non-traumatic cerebrospinal rhinorrhoea. *Acta Neurol Scand* 1982; 66: 180–192.

13. Weisberg LA. Housepain EM, Saur DP. Empty sella syndrome as a complication of benign intracranial hypertension. *J Neurosurg* 1977; 43: 177–180.

14. Dlouhy BJ, Madhavan K, Clinger JD, et al. Elevated body mass index and risk of postoperative CSF leak following transsphenoidal surgery. *J Neurosurg* 2012; 116(6): 1311–1317. doi: 10.3171/2012.2.JNS111837

15. Berdahl JP, Fleischman D, Zaydlarova J, et al. Body mass index has a linear relationship with cerebrospinal fluid pressure. *Invest Ophthalmol Vis Sci* 2012; 53: 1422–1427.

16. Jennum P, Borgesen SE. Intracranial pressure and obstructive sleep apnea. *Chest* 1989; 95: 279–283.

17. Pérez MA, Bialer OY, Bruce BB, et al. Primary spontaneous cerebrospinal fluid leaks and idiopathic intracranial hypertension. *J Neuroophthalmol* 2013; 33(4): 330–337. doi: 10.1097/WNO.0b013e318299c292

18. Corbett JJ, Savino PJ, Thompson HS, et al. Visual loss in pseudotumor cerebri. Follow-up of 57 patients from five to 41 years and a profile of 14 patients with permanent severe visual loss. *Arch Neurol* 1982; 39: 461–474.

19. Ball AK, Howman A, Wheatley K, et al. A randomised controlled trial of treatment for idiopathic intracranial hypertension. *J Neurol* 2011; 258: 874–881.

20. Corbett JJ, Mehta MP. Cerebrospinal fluid pressure in normal obese subjects and patients with pseudotumor cerebri. *Neurology* 1983; 33: 1386–1388.

21. Wang EW, Vandergrift WA 3rd, Schlosser RJ. Spontaneous CSF leaks. *Otolaryngol Clinics North Am* 2011; 44: 845–856.

22. Schlosser RJ, Bolger WE. Significance of empty sella in cerebrospinal fluid leaks. *Otolaryngol Head Neck Surg* 2003; 128: 32–38.

23. Silver RI, Moonis G, Schlosser RJ, Bolger WE, Loevner LA. Radiographic signs of elevated intracranial pressure in idiopathic cerebrospinal fluid leaks: A possible presentation of idiopathic intracranial hypertension. *Am J Rhinol* 2007; 21: 257–261.

24. Butros SR, Goncalves LF, Thompson D, Agarwal A, Lee HK. Imaging features of idiopathic intracranial hypertension, including a new finding: Widening of the foramen ovale. *Acta Radiol* 2012; 53: 682–688.

25. Shetty PG, Shroff MM, Fatterpekar GM, Sahani DV, Kirtane MV. A retrospective analysis of spontaneous sphenoid sinus fistula: MR and CT findings. *Am J Neuroradiol* 2000; 21: 337–342.

26. Psaltis AJ, Overton LJ, Thomas WW III, et al. Differences in skull base thickness in patients with spontaneous cerebrospinal fluid leaks. *Am J Rhinol Allergy* 2014; 28:e73–e79.

27. Schlosser RJ, Bolger WE. Spontaneous nasal cerebrospinal fluid leaks and empty sella syndrome: A clinical association. *Am J Rhinol* 2003; 17: 91–96.

28. Miller NR. Pseudotumor cerebri, In Winn HR (Ed.), *Youmans Neurological Surgery* (5 ed.). Philadelphia, PA: WB Saunders, 2003, Vol. 1, pp. 1419–1434.

29. Newborg B. Pseudotumor cerebri treated by rice/reduction diet. *Arch Intern Med* 1974; 133: 802–807.

30. Jacobson DM, Berg R, Wall M, et al. Serum vitamin A concentration is elevated in idiopathic intracranial hypertension. *Neurology* 1999; 53: 1114–1118.

31. Friedman DI, Ingram P, Rogers MAM. Low tyramine diet in the treatment of idiopathic intracranial hypertension: A pilot study. *Neurology* 1998; 50: A5.

32. Chan JW. Current concepts and strategies in the diagnosis and management of idiopathic intracranial hypertension in adults. *J Neurol* 2017; 264: 1622–1633.

33. Wall M. Idiopathic intracranial hypertension (pseudotumor cerebri). *Curr Neurol Neurosci Rep* 2008; 8: 87–93.

34. Corbett JJ, Thompson HS. The rational management of idiopathic intracranial hypertension. *Arch Neurol* 1989; 46: 1049–1051.

35. Aaron G, Doyle J, Vaphiades MS, et al. Increased intracranial pressure in spontaneous CSF leak patients is not associated with papilledema. *Otolaryngol Head Neck Surg* 2014; 151(6): 1061–1066. doi: 10.1177/0194599814551122

36. Keltner JL. Optic nerve sheath decompression. How does it work? Has its time come? *Arch Ophthalmol* 1988; 106: 1365–1369.

37. Ngyun R, Carta A, Geleris A, et al. Long-term effect of optic nerve sheath decompression on intracranial pressure in pseudotumor cerebri. *Invest Ophth Vis Sci* 1997; 38: S388.

38. Mittra RA, Sergott RC, Flaharty PM, et al. Optic nerve decompression improves hemodynamic parameters in papilledema. *Ophthalmology* 1993; 100: 987–97.

39. Dinkin MJ, Patsalides A. Venous sinus stenting for idiopathic intracranial hypertension: Where are we now? *Neurol Clin* 2017; 35: 59–81.
40. Higgins JN, Owler BK, Cousins C, Pickard JD. Venous sinus stenting for refractory benign intracranial hypertension. *Lancet* 2002; 359: 228–230.
41. Starke RM, Wang T, Ding D, et al. Endovascular treatment of venous sinus stenosis in idiopathic intracranial hypertension: Complications, neurological outcomes, and radiographic results. *Sci World J* 2015; 2015: 140408.
42. Elder BD, Rory Goodwin C, Kosztowski TA, et al. Venous sinus stenting is a valuable treatment for fulminant idiopathic intracranial hypertension. *J Clin Neurosci* 2015; 22: 685–689.
43. Puffer RC, Mustafa W, Lanzino G. Venous sinus stenting for idiopathic intracranial hypertension: A review of the literature. *J Neurointerv Surg* 2013; 5: 483–486.
44. Ahmed RM, Wilkinson M, Parker GD, et al. Transverse sinus stenting for idiopathic intracranial hypertension: A review of 52 patients and of model predictions. *Am J Neuroradiol* 2011; 32: 1408–1414.
45. Teleb MS, Cziep ME, Lazzaro MA, et al. Idiopathic intracranial hypertension. A systematic analysis of transverse sinus stenting. *Interv Neurol* 2013; 2: 132–143.
46. Xu K, Yu T, Yuan Y, Yu J. Current status of the application of intracranial venous sinus stenting. *Int J Med Sci* 2015; 12: 780–789.
47. Radvany MG, Solomon D, Nijjar S, et al. Visual and neurological outcomes following endovascular stenting for pseudotumor cerebri associated with transverse sinus stenosis. *J Neuroophthalmol* 2013; 33: 117–122.
48. Fields JD, Javedani PP, Falardeau J, et al. Dural venous sinus angioplasty and stenting for the treatment of idiopathic intracranial hypertension. *J Neurointerv Surg* 2013; 5: 62–68.
49. Owler BK, Parker G, Halmagyi GM, et al. Pseudotumor cerebri syndrome: Venous sinus obstruction and its treatment with stent placement. *J Neurosurg* 2003; 98: 1045–1055.
50. Satti SR, Leishangthem L, Chaudry MI. Meta-analysis of CSF diversion procedures and dural venous sinus stenting in the setting of medically refractory idiopathic intracranial hypertension. *Am J Neuroradiol* 2015; 36: 1899–1904.
51. Campbell RG, Farquhar D, Zhao N, et al. Cerebrospinal fluid rhinorrhea secondary to idiopathic intracranial hypertension: Long-term outcomes of endoscopic repairs. *Am J Rhinol Allergy* 2016; 30: 294–300. doi: 10.2500/ajra.2016.30.4319

# 8

# Systemic causes of CSF rhinorrhea

HEMANTH VAMANSHANKAR AND JYOTIRMAY S HEGDE

CSF rhinorrhea may be associated with a variety of systemic disorders. In many cases, CSF rhinorrhea may be the first clinical symptom of a genetic disorder, especially those associated with hereditary disorders of connective tissues. Most of these manifestations may be diagnosed clinically. Hence, a thorough history and detailed general physical and local examination of various systems of the body have to be undertaken in cases of spontaneous CSF rhinorrhea. This is of great importance, as the underlying factor for the cause of CSF rhinorrhea has to be found and first treated before undertaking a formal closure of the CSF leak. This may reduce the chance of recurrences and associated complications in these cases, thus preventing the possibility of a second procedure and morbidity to the patient.

## MORNING GLORY SYNDROME

A rare congenital abnormality first described by Kindler in 1970.[1] It is due to the failure of closure of embryonic choroid fissure. Presentation is usually unilateral, with loss/ impaired vision, hypertelorism, strabismus and leukocoria. Fundoscopic examination reveals a funnel-shaped optic nerve head with a central white point of glial tissue surrounded by an elevated annulus of chorioretinal pigment disturbance, thus giving the appearance of a morning glory flower[2,3] (Figures 8.1 and 8.2). Other abnormalities associated with morning glory syndrome are cleft palate, hypopituitarism, mental retardation, and agenesis of the

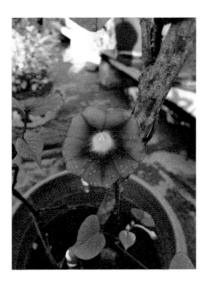

Figure 8.1 Morning glory flower. © Jyotirmay S Hegde, Hemanth Vamanshankar.

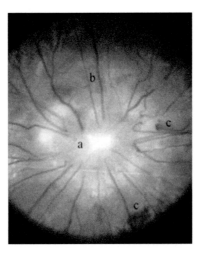

Figure 8.2 Fundoscopic picture of patient with morning glory syndrome (a) funnel-shaped optic disc; (b) radiating retinal vessels; (c) pigmented peripapillar tissue. (Photograph printed with permission from Ref. 4).

corpus callosum. This syndrome is seen in 67.7% of basal encephaloceles (another rare entity seen in 1:35000 live births).[4] Spontaneous CSF rhinorrhea is the usual presentation in cases of basal encephaloceles.

## EHLERS-DANLOS SYNDROME (EDS)

Two subtypes have been described:[5-7]

1. Ehlers-Danlos syndrome classic type: Characterized by joint hypermobility and extensive skin involvement: skin hyperextensibility, abnormal wound healing, and scar formation. Fragility of other connective tissues is also noted, causing cervical insufficiency in pregnancy, recurrent hernias, and rectal prolapse. Cauliflower deformity of skin collagen fibrils on histology is characteristic of the classic type of EDS. Diagnosis is usually clinical, but almost 50% have mutations of the COL5A1 or COL5A2 gene. However, a negative test cannot rule out its absence.
2. Ehlers-Danlos syndrome hypermobility type: This is the more common subtype of EDS. It presents with chronic painful instability of joints associated with joint dislocations. This further leads to degenerative joint disease in young adults. Skin involvement, however, is mild: soft skin that bruises easily. The genetic basis of this subtype is unknown. A positive family history may sometimes be elicited in these patients. Diagnosis is clinical.

Reinstein et al. have reported six cases of Ehlers-Danlos syndrome patients (four hypermobility type and two classic types) with a history of spontaneous CSF leaks. They report the prevalence of such hereditary connective tissue disorders as 1:5000 live births.[8]

## MARFAN SYNDROME

Mutation of the gene FBN1 is present in this type of hereditary connective tissue disorder in >95% patients. Skeletal manifestations include a marfanoid habitus, scoliosis, pectus carinatum, joint pains, high arched palate, malar hypoplasia, and retrognathia. Ocular defects include lens dislocation, bilateral retinal detachment, and myopia. Aortic root dilatation is seen as a cardiovascular manifestation. CSF leaks from the dural sac have been reported in this condition.[8]

## BENIGN JOINT HYPERMOBILITY SYNDROME (BJHM) AND ISOLATED CONNECTIVE TISSUE DISORDERS (ICTD)

BJHM patients present in the spectrum of hereditary disorders of connective tissue with joint laxity and a familial incidence of hypermobility. However, no skin involvement is noted in these patients. ICTD patients present with mild craniofacial findings. Both these disorders have reported associated spontaneous CSF leaks.[8]

Systemic manifestations which are seen in hereditary connective tissue disorders are listed in Table 8.1. It is imperative to check other systems in an isolated case of spontaneous CSF rhinorrhea so as to rule out systemic causes.

## CRANIOFACIAL DYSOSTOSES – CROUZON SYNDROME

Crouzon syndrome is an autosomal dominant syndrome caused by mutation in the gene encoding for fibroblast growth factor receptor 2 on chromosome 10. It presents as a triad of midface hypoplasia, exophthalmos, and premature craniosynostosis. 63% of these are predisposed to have an elevated intracranial pressure. Further complications of Crouzon syndrome like hydrocephalus, obstructive sleep apnoea, and intracranial venous congestion also contribute to raised intracranial pressure. The proposed mechanism of leaks in these patients is due to persistent intracranial hypertension. This causes inferior displacement of cribriform plates and thinning of the anterior cranial base, thus facilitating the formation of a fistula and leak. Also, surgical corrections in Crouzon syndrome by a high-level nasal frontoethmoidal osteotomy (due to unreliable markers of craniofacial bony anatomy) may be predisposed to tearing of the anterior cranial base dura and CSF leak.[9]

## ALBERS-SCHÖNBERG DISEASE

An autosomal dominant sclerosing disorder of the skeletal system, characterized by increased bone density caused by heterozygous mutations in the chloride channel 7 gene. High-pressure leak secondary to a hydrocephalus in this congenital anomaly has been described.[10]

## ENDOCRINE ABNORMALITIES

Isolated cases of hypo/hyperadrenalism, hypothyroidism with myxedema and hypoparathyroidism have seen to be associated with increased CSF pressure and papilledema. These have in turn been implicated as rare causes of pseudotumor cerebri and spontaneous CSF leaks. The pathological basis of why increased CSF pressure and papilledema develop is not known.[11]

## TAKE-HOME POINTS

- Spontaneous CSF rhinorrhea may be the first symptom in these systemic conditions.
- Detailed history and general examination are of utmost importance in diagnosis.
- Treatment of the systemic factor(s) should be undertaken prior to treating the CSF leak.

Table 8.1  Associated systemic manifestations seen in hereditary connective tissue disorders[8]

| Dermatologic | Orthopedic | Cardiovascular | Craniofacial | Obstetric/ Gynecological | Ophthalmologic |
|---|---|---|---|---|---|
| • Skin hyperextensibility/ elasticity<br>• Thin and soft, transparent skin<br>• Stretch marks<br>• Widened scars<br>• Slow wound healing<br>• Easy bruising, ecchymoses | • Joint hypermobility<br>• Degenerative joint disease<br>• Scoliosis<br>• Chronic limb and joint pains<br>• Joint dislocation<br>• Fractures<br>• Flat feet | • Aortic aneurysm/ rupture/dissection<br>• Valvular disease (esp. mitral valve prolapse). | • Dental crowding<br>• Dysmorphic faces<br>• High arched palate<br>• Single/bifid uvula | • Uterine rupture/ cervical insufficiency during pregnancy<br>• Pregnancy associated maternal complications | • Lens dislocation<br>• Retinal detachment<br>• Blue sclera<br>• Vision abnormalities |

# REFERENCES

1. Kindler P. Morning glory syndrome: Unusual congenital optic disk anomaly. *Am J Ophthalmol* 1970; 69:376–84.
2. Lit ES, D'Amico DJ. Retinal manifestations of morning glory disc syndrome. *Int Ophthalmol Clin* 2001; 41:131–8.
3. Soyer P, Dobbelaere P, Benoit S. Transalar sphenoidal encephalocele. Uncommon clinical and radiological findings. *Clin Radiol* 1991; 43:65–7.
4. Sasani M, Ozer AF, Aydin AL. Endoscopic treatment of trans-sellar trans-sphenoidal encephalocele associated with morning glory syndrome presenting with non-traumatic cerebrospinal fluid rhinorrhea. *J Neurosurg Sci* 2009; 53:31–5.
5. Castori M, Camerota F, Celletti C, Grammatico P, Padua L. Natural history and manifestations of the hypermobility type Ehlers-Danlos syndrome: A pilot study on 21 patients. *Am J Med Genet A* 2010; 152:556–564.
6. Beighton P, De Paepe A, Steinmann B, Tsipouras P, Wenstrup RJ. Ehlers-Danlos syndromes: Revised nosology, villefranche, 1997. *Am J Med Genet* 1998; 77:31–7.
7. Malfait F, Wenstrup RJ, De Paepe A. Clinical and genetic aspects of Ehlers-Danlos syndrome, classic type. *Genet Med* 2010; 12:597–605.
8. Reinstein E, Pariani M, Bannykh S, Rimoin DL, Schievink WI. Connective tissue spectrum abnormalities associated with spontaneous cerebrospinal fluid leaks: A prospective study. *Eur J Hum Gen* 2013; 21:386–390.
9. Panuganti BA, Leach M, Antisdel J. Bilateral meningoencephaloceles with cerebrospinal fluid rhinorrhea after facial advancement in the Crouzon syndrome. *Allergy Rhinol.* 2015; 6(2):138–142.
10. Ommaya AK, Chiro G D, Baldwin M, Pennybacker JB. Non-traumatic cerebrospinal fluid rhinorrhoea. *J Neurol Neurosurg Psychiat* 1968; 31:214–225.
11. Allan HR, Robert HB. Chapter 30: Disturbances of cerebrospinal fluid and its circulation. In *Adam's and Victor's Principles of Neurology* (8th ed.). New York, NY: McGraw Hill, 2005, p. 540.

# 9

# Endoscopic management of CSF rhinorrhea

JYOTIRMAY S HEGDE AND HEMANTH VAMANSHANKAR

The management of CSF rhinorrhea resulting from defects in the skull base depends on several factors like site, size, access, underlying cause, and the general condition of the patient. The introduction of endoscopes for minimally invasive endonasal approaches for CSF leak repair has revolutionized treatment for many patients. A transnasal approach to sphenoid sinus leaks was reported by

Hirsch using septal flaps in 1952. Vrabec and Hallberg described an intranasal approach for cribriform plate leaks in 1964. The use of endoscopes for the repair of small CSF leaks occurring during ethmoidectomy began only in 1981 and was popularized by Wigand. Since then, there has been a lot of progress in the endoscopic approach to the management of CSF rhinorrhea. However, the endoscopic approach has its own limitations and may not be applicable in all cases.

Our protocol for the endoscopic management of CSF rhinorrhea:

A. Diagnosis of CSF leak
B. Localization of the site of leak
C. Medical management
D. Surgical management; site-specific management of the leak
E. Post-operative management

## DIAGNOSIS OF A CSF LEAK

Beta-2 transferrin immunofixation is currently the biochemical investigation of choice for diagnosing CSF rhinorrhea. It is found in CSF, vitreous fluid of the eye, and the perilymph. It has a high sensitivity and specificity of 100% and 71% respectively for the detection of CSF leaks.[1] It was first introduced by Meurman et al. in 1979.[2] The disadvantages are that it is an expensive test and it is usually outsourced in most hospitals with a turnaround time of 5–7 days.

Beta trace protein ($\beta$-TP): $\beta$-TP is another diagnostic marker for CSF rhinorrhea. It has been used as a low cost, non-invasive test. It is one of the most abundant proteins in CSF, and is present in other body fluids at a much lower concentration. The assay requires a small sample size (200 $\mu$L) and results can be obtained within 20 minutes. It has a similar sensitivity and specificity to $\beta$2-transferrin assays.[3] It is unreliable in the presence of renal disease and meningitis.[4]

Glucose oxidase: The CSF glucose concentration typically exceeds serum concentration by 50%.[5] Analysis of glucose concentration in nasal secretions suspicious for CSF has therefore been used since the late 1800s. It has high false-positive and negative rates due to many reasons including hyperglycaemia, bacterial contamination, and even excessive assay sensitivity.[6] Glucose oxidase testing is currently of historical value only.[3]

## LOCALIZATION OF THE SITE OF LEAK

Diagnostic nasal endoscopy: Localization of the dural defect should be attempted after confirmation of CSF rhinorrhea with diagnostic testing. Nasal endoscopy can be used to localize the side or general location of the leak. However, visualization of the actual fistula site is often challenging or difficult in routine cases.[3]

High-resolution computed tomography (HRCT) scan: The gold standard for localization of CSF rhinorrhoea is by HRCT. It non-invasive, inexpensive, and has a sensitivity of approximately 87% for the identification of CSF rhinorrhea.[7] The cribriform and sphenoethmoid defects are better identified in coronal

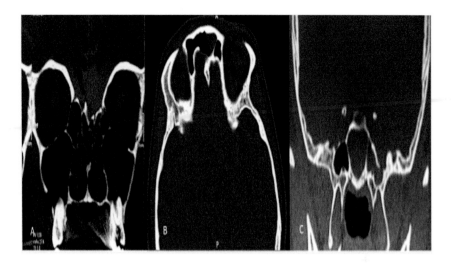

Figure 9.1 CT scan A – CT scan showing defect in the left cribriform plate and fovea. CT scan B – CT scan showing defect in the posterior table of right frontal sinus. CT scan C – CT scan showing defect in the lateral recess of left sphenoid sinus. © Jyotirmay S Hegde, Hemanth Vamanshankar.

images, while identification of posterior table, frontal sinus defects are appreciated well in axial and sagittal cuts[8] (Figures 9.1, 9.2).

CT cisternography: CT cisternography is usually used as an adjunct to high-resolution CT for active CSF drainage. An intrathecal injection of approximately 3–10 mL, of an iodinated non-ionic low-osmolar contrast agent is performed.

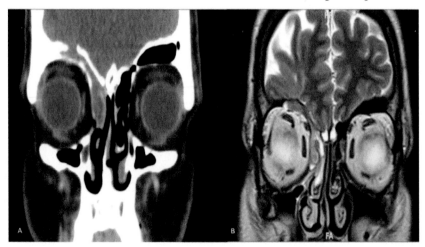

Figure 9.2 Comparison of CT and MRI findings showing defect in the posterior wall of the frontal sinus. A CT scan showing defect in the posterior table of right frontal sinus. B MRI scan showing defect in the posterior table of right frontal sinus. © Jyotirmay S Hegde, Hemanth Vamanshankar.

The patient is positioned in a Trendelenburg position to opacify the basal cisterns or prone with the head in the dependent position. It has a sensitivity of 80–95%.[4,9] It has high sensitivity in frontal or sphenoid sinus leaks, because these sinuses act as reservoirs to collect the contrast material. Leaks from cribriform and ethmoid areas can drain more readily into the nasopharynx and may be difficult to identify by CT cisternography.[10] CT cisternography is a minimally invasive procedure, but the limitations are headache, meningeal irritation, and seizures and the disadvantage is its need for an active CSF leak.[11]

Magnetic resonance imaging (MRI): MRI is a useful adjunct for localizing CSF leaks. CSF is hyper-intense on T2-weighted imaging and can be readily identified within the nasal cavity.[9] It also provides higher resolution of the soft tissues for identification of brain/dural herniations. It can achieve a sensitivity of 85–92% and specificity of nearly 100%.[10] MRI is, however, more time-consuming, costly, and physically more difficult to obtain (due to gantry size and patient tolerance). Hence, MRI is more of an adjunct to HRCT (Figures 9.3, 9.4).

Magnetic resonance cisternogram (MRC): The principle of MR cisternography is to demonstrate a contiguous fluid signal between the cisternal space and nasal sinus on heavily weighted T2 images. Magnetic resonance cisternography is performed with an intrathecal injection of contrast material via lumbar puncture. The detection of CSF within the nasal cavity can be enhanced with this method. The risk of neurological changes or seizure activity with the use of gadolinium is extremely low.[12] The sensitivity is approximately 85–92% and specificity of 100% with MRC.[10] Magnetic resonance cisternography is expensive and more time-consuming than high-resolution CT. The limitations are headache, meningeal irritation, seizures, and its need for an active CSF leak.

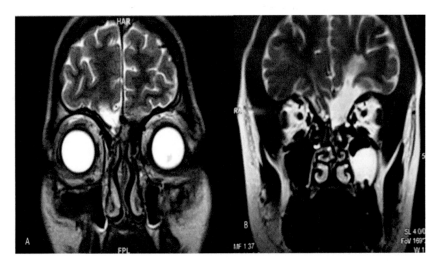

Figure 9.3 A – MRI scan depicting defect in the right cribriform plate. B – MRI scan depicting defect in the left fovea ethmoidalis. © Jyotirmay S Hegde, Hemanth Vamanshankar.

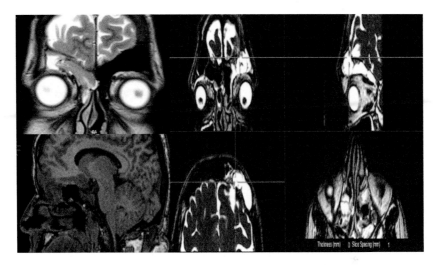

Figure 9.4 MRI scans showing defect in various planes. © Jyotirmay S Hegde, Hemanth Vamanshankar.

Radionucleotide cisternogram: This technique involves intrathecal injection of a radioactive isotope via lumbar puncture. Radionuclide cisternography is performed with a radiotracer: technetium (Tc) 99m-labeled diethylenetriamine penta-acetic acid for active CSF leaks, which has a short half-life of about 6 hours. Intermittent CSF leaks are demonstrated by a prolonged cisternography, which can be performed with a radiotracer: Indium (In) 111-labeled diethylenetriamine penta-acetic acid, which has a longer half-life with delayed imaging of up to 72 hrs. The sensitivity of the test is only 62–76%.[13]

Intrathecal fluorescein: Intrathecal fluorescein is used almost exclusively for localization of CSF leaks in the intraoperative setting (Figure 9.5).

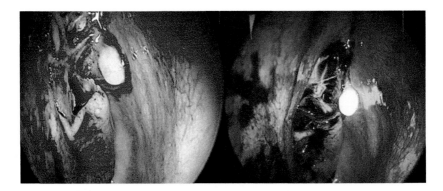

Figure 9.5 Fluoroscein stained defect with and without blue-green filter before repair. © Jyotirmay S Hegde, Hemanth Vamanshankar.

# MEDICAL MANAGEMENT

These include the following:

- Elevation of the head end of bed to around 30 degrees, avoidance of straining and routine use of stool softeners are usually employed in medical management. The majority of the post-traumatic CSF rhinorrhea resolve with a medical line of management. Bell et al. found resolution of CSF leaks in 85% of the patients in a review of 34 cases of traumatic skull base CSF rhinorrhea treated by medical management.[14] Raised ICP (intracranial pressure) could be one of the reasons for persistent leak. Carbonic anhydrase inhibitors like acetazolamide, which act by decreasing secretion of CSF from choroid plexus is accepted as the first line treatment in lowering ICP. Diuretics like furosemide, spironolactone and triamterene have also been used. Corticosteroids may be used in the short term for the rapid decrease of ICP as an adjunct surgical management. Benign intracranial hypertension and its management has been dealt in detail in Chapter 7. Around 68% of the post-traumatic CSF leaks closed spontaneously within 48 hours and 85% closed within 7 days of initial injury in a study done by Mincy.[15]
- CSF diversion for 7–10 days can help in treating persistent CSF rhinorrhea. A lumbar drain is the most commonly used technique. However, in patients with traumatic brain injury or those requiring intracranial pressure monitoring may need an external ventriculostomy.[16,17] Pressure can be reduced by optimal CSF drainage (10 mL/hour) without resulting in CSF hypovolemia.[18] CSF diversion as an adjunct to medical management raises the success rate to approximately 90%.[14] CSF diversion is also used as part of routine postoperative management after repair of skull base defects, especially in the case of high-pressure leaks.
- Prophylactic antibiotics: The most common major complication associated with posttraumatic CSF rhinorrhea is meningitis. There is a 0.62% chance of meningitis in the first 24 hours, 9.12% after a week, and 18.82% after 2 weeks as per a study undertaken by Eljamel and Foy. The use of routine prophylactic antibiotics in patients with skull base fractures to reduce the risk of meningitis is doubtful, according to a Cochrane review.[19]

# SURGICAL MANAGEMENT

## Peri-operative issues

### PLACEMENT OF LUMBAR DRAIN AND INTRATHECAL FLUORESCEIN

A lumbar drain is placed before beginning the surgical approach. It can be difficult to identify the subarachnoid space and withdraw CSF or place the lumbar drain in patients with a high-volume CSF leak. It is easy to place the lumbar drain with the patient awake and in a sitting position to fill the lumbar cistern with CSF. The other option is to place the lumbar drain after intubation and elevate the head of the bed to assist in dilating the lumbar cistern with CSF.[20]

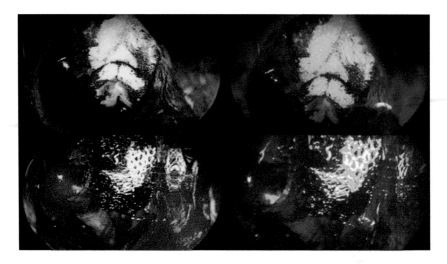

Figure 9.6 Fluoroscein stained defect with and without blue-green filter after repair. © Jyotirmay S Hegde, Hemanth Vamanshankar.

0.1 mL of 10% fluorescein solution is diluted in 10 mL of CSF and is injected slowly into the intrathecal space through the spinal needle over 10 minutes. Fluorescein helps in precise identification of the bony skull base defect and CSF leak (Figure 9.6). Complications are usually related to higher concentrations, more rapid injections, or suboccipital punctures.[21] The lumbar catheter is inserted, secured, and clamped for the initial part of the surgery.

Around 10 to 15 mL of CSF is removed over 15 minutes, once the skull base defect is exposed to aid in reduction of the cauterized encephalocele base. The lumbar drain is kept open after graft placement, draining 5 to 10 mL of CSF per hour for the remainder of the procedure and for the initial postoperative period. The height of the drain is adjusted to keep the drainage between 5 and 10 mL of CSF per hour.[20]

The lumbar drain is very useful in avoiding a rise in ICP if the patient coughs or strains during the perioperative period or has nausea and vomiting during the immediate postoperative period. The lumbar drain is clamped for 6 to 12 hours to ensure leak cessation and removed between the 3rd and 5th postoperative day. The lumbar drain can be reopened for 2 to 3 days, or the patient is taken for surgical re-exploration if there is a CSF leak on clamping the drain.

## NASAL PACKING

The nostril is packed with cotton pledgets soaked in 4% Xylocaine with adrenaline.

## ANTIBIOTICS

The use of perioperative antibiotics is routinely followed before repair of a CSF leak, as tissue grafts are placed through the contaminated or colonized nasal cavity to rest against brain tissue at the skull base defect and risk an infection of the central nervous system. It is advisable to use intravenous ceftriaxone because of its CSF penetration. The other alternatives that afford a degree of blood-brain barrier penetration and can be helpful in patients with cephalosporin allergies are trimethoprim-sulfamethoxazole and levofloxacin. In addition, antibiotic solution (clindamycin) irrigation of the nasal cavity may be done in an attempt to minimize bacterial contamination.[20]

## VACCINATION

Patients undergoing elective repair of CSF rhinorrhea should be evaluated for pneumococcal antibody titers. In the case of low values, they should ideally be vaccinated with 23-valent polysaccharide pneumococcal vaccine or 7-valent conjugate pneumococcal vaccine.

## POSITIVE PRESSURE VENTILATION

Positive pressure ventilation carries a high risk of pneumocephalus. Hence, while administering anesthesia, it is advisable to perform rapid sequence intubation and minimize masking the patient and using positive-pressure ventilation.

# Surgical approach

## SITE-SPECIFIC MANAGEMENT OF THE LEAK

1. Cribriform plate and ethmoid roof
2. Sphenoid sinus, lateral recess of sphenoid and perisellar regions
3. Frontal sinus
4. Multiple sites of leak

1. Cribriform plate and ethmoid roof

   A routine transnasal endoscopic approach is used to treat leaks in the cribriform plate and ethmoid roof. The nose is decongested first with topical vasoconstrictors and then irrigated with antibiotic solution to reduce bacteria within the surgical field and reduce the potential for intracranial complications. The defects localized in the medial lamella of the cribriform plate can be repaired under direct visualization (Figure 9.7).

   For defects involving the lateral lamella of the cribriform plate and fovea ethmoidalis, middle meatal antrostomy and ethmoidectomy are usually needed to provide adequate exposure of the skull base defect and leak. Middle and/or superior turbinectomies are performed if additional exposure is needed. Frontal and sphenoid sinus ostial widening is done in addition if required, in order to prevent mucoceles (Video 4).

2. Sphenoid sinus, lateral recess of sphenoid and perisellar regions

   Sphenoid defects can be approached through the medial, intermediate, and lateral approaches. Posterior septectomy may be done for additional exposure of the midline perisellar or clival regions. Defects located in the lateral recess of the sphenoid sinus may require an endoscopic transpterygoid approach.[22]

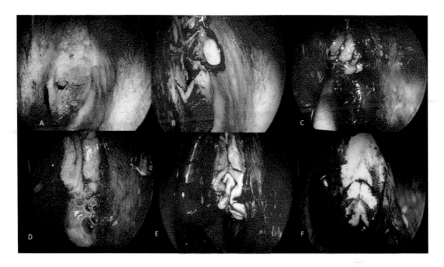

Figure 9.7 A to F showing various phases of CSF leak repair in the right cribriform plate. © Jyotirmay S Hegde, Hemanth Vamanshankar.

A wide middle meatal antrostomy, anterior and posterior ethmoidectomy and wide sphenoidotomy are performed. Then the pterygopalatine fossa is entered after the posterior wall of the maxillary sinus is removed. The internal maxillary artery and its branches are identified, moved inferiorly, or clipped and divided to expose the deeper areas of the pterygopalatine fossa. The sphenopalatine ganglion, vidian nerve and V2 are dissected free, and preserved if possible. The pterygoid plate is drilled or curetted away to gain access to the lateral recess of the sphenoid sinus[20] (Video 5).

3. Frontal sinus

Frontal sinus CSF leaks generally can be either near the frontal recess, in the frontal recess proper, or the posterior table of frontal sinus. It may be difficult to access anatomically because of the angulation. Hence it may necessitate the use of angled scopes, frontal trephining, or a combined endoscopic and external approach, depending on the site of the leak.

The CSF leaks which are located near the frontal recess but do not involve the frontal sinus or its outflow tract directly are managed by a purely endonasal endoscopic approach. The frontal recess is opened to avoid iatrogenic mucoceles and the defect is closed after visualization of the leak site. The defects that directly involve the frontal recess may require either an isolated endoscopic approach or a minimal-access combined endoscopic and external approach (MACA), depending on the extent of the defect. The defects involving the posterior table above the isthmus of the frontal recess may be managed by an advanced endoscopic approach, frontal trephination and an endoscopic-modified Lothrop procedure. However, defects which are located superiorly or laterally within the frontal sinus still may require an osteoplastic flap with or without obliteration. The specific approach depends on the site and size of the defect, the equipment available, and surgical experience.[20]

The standard approach for CSF repair for leaks around the frontal recess include uncinectomy, middle meatal antrostomy, followed by removal of agar nasi and frontal cells. Next, the frontal recess and ostium are identified, followed by identification of the site of the leak. Care should be taken while repairing the defect to prevent blockage of the frontal recess and ostium.

Extended endoscopic approach or frontal trephination or the minimal access combined approach may be required for defects which involve the lateral part of the frontal sinus or the posterior table of the frontal sinus.

An extended endoscopic approach involves the Draf type IIb or type III procedure and the bi-nostril approach by using the contralateral nasal fossa, the orbital transposition obtained by drilling out the superomedial bony wall of the orbit and the use of double-curved instruments to the far lateral aspect of the frontal sinus and/or the supraorbital recess in selected cases.[23]

Frontal sinus trephination is preferred in cases in which an open osteoplastic flap procedure is too aggressive and a purely endoscopic approach is not feasible. The infrabrow incision is the most common approach and is located at the superomedial aspect of the orbit, medial to the supraorbital neurovascular bundle, and immediately below the eyebrow and supraorbital rim.[24]

The MACA is ideal in repairing the defects that directly involve the frontal recess because the superior extent of the defect may be difficult to reach endoscopically, and the inferior/posterior/medial/lateral extension of the defect may be difficult to reach from an external approach. The infrabrow incision similar to the one used during frontal trephination is used to approach the frontal sinus (Figure 9.8). The skin incision is around 1–2 cm, terminating at the medial brow. The incision is carried through the periosteum and the deeper tissues. The periosteum is elevated using freers or a periosteum elevator to expose the underlying bone. The exact point of frontal sinus penetration is marked in or near the floor the frontal sinus. It can be navigation guided if facilities are available. A 4 mm round cutting/diamond burr is used to perform the external trephination. The window is widened using a Kerrison rongeur sufficient to accommodate an endoscope and an instrument. The frontal trephination can be combined with an endoscopic frontal sinusotomy using a minimal access-combined external and endoscopic approach technique (Video 1).

4. Multiple sites of leak

Multiple defects may be visualized in the same patient and need to be addressed appropriately (Figure 9.9). The underlying etiology is usually traumatic in nature but may be also seen in cases of leaks secondary to benign intracranial hypertension or hypothyroidism. If the defects are multiple and difficult to be addressed endoscopically, they should be managed by a transcranial route. Intrathecal fluorescein and image guided navigation also aids in the visualization and confirmation of multiple defects (Video 3).

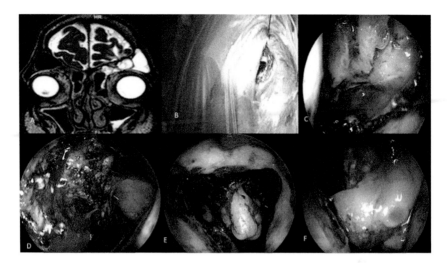

Figure 9.8  A – MRI showing defect in the posterior table of frontal sinus. B – Left infrabrow incision. C – Defect in the posterior table of frontal sinus with the meningocele. D – Cauterization of the encephalocele with mucosal removal of the margins. E – Reconstruction of defect with fat. F – Reconstruction of defect with fascia lata and glue. © Jyotirmay S Hegde, Hemanth Vamanshankar.

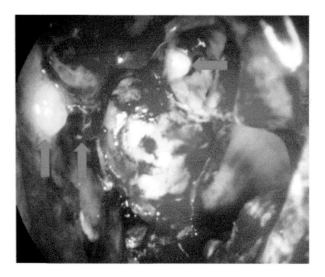

Figure 9.9  Showing multiple defects (blue arrows) in the right skull base with help of intrathecal fluorescein. © Jyotirmay S Hegde, Hemanth Vamanshankar.

## Contraindications to an endoscopic approach

Not all cases are suitable or indicated for endoscopic repair. The following are a few of the contraindications in the current scenario[20]

1. Multiple, comminuted fracture of the skull base
2. CSF leaks associated with tumors
3. High-pressure leaks requiring CSF diversion procedures
4. Large skull base defects
5. Badly deformed skull bases

Cases not suitable for endoscopic approach are dealt with by an intracranial approach. This has been dealt with detail in Chapter 10.

We have described our protocol in the management of CSF rhinorrhea (Figure 9.10).

## Endoscopic repair technique

The stereotactic image guidance system is ensured to be in proper working order and properly calibrated in case it is used. Thorough endoscopic examination of the suspected area of leak is undertaken, and seen for areas of meningoencephalocele, mucosal edema as a result of long-standing exposure to CSF or for areas of yellow-green fluorescein. The navigation system can be used at this juncture to confirm the site of leak and its proximity to the vital structures. The meningoencephalocele is reduced using bipolar cautery. The mucosa surrounding the defect is removed or debrided to create the recipient bed and to avoid secretion from sinus mucosa. It is very important to remove the mucosa thoroughly to expose the underlying bone. A diamond burr or curette can be used to abrade the recipient bed bone lightly and stimulate osteoneogenesis once adequate mucosa is removed. Monopolar cautery should be avoided near or adjacent to the lamina papyracea, optic nerve, or carotid arteries to avoid complications like blindness or uncontrollable bleeding. Bi-polar cautery is used to control any bleeding around the defect meticulously, especially when near the base of the encephalocele to avoid intracranial hemorrhage. The lumbar drain is opened and CSF is diverted away from the graft site when the base of the encephalocele is being cauterized, in order to facilitate graft placement.[20]

The size of the bony defect is measured approximately to plan the reconstruction of the defect. The reconstruction plan depends on the site, size, and etiology of the defect. Another important factor which decides the success of the closure is the underlying intracranial pressure (ICP).[25] The reconstruction is done by underlay, overlay or a combination of an underlay and overlay technique. Grafts, flaps, and adjuvants are used in reconstruction of the defect. Grafts can be autologous, acellular human dermis, or engineered collagen. Flaps can be pedicled or free flaps. Adjuvants can be rigid support (natural or synthetic) or tissue glues.

Based on maximum diameter of defects, those which are 2.5 cm or less are termed minor defects, while those greater than 2.5 cm diameter are major defects.[26]

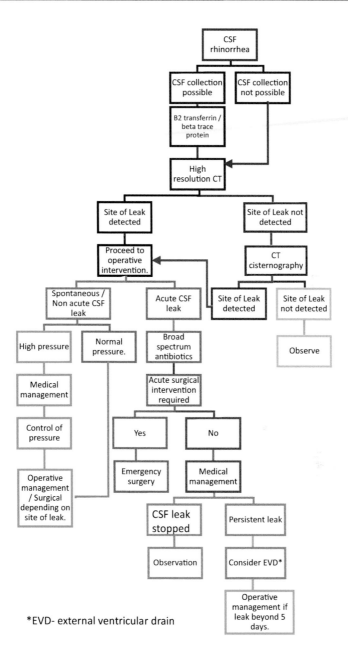

Figure 9.10 Flowchart depicting our protocol in the management of CSF rhinorrhea. © Jyotirmay S Hegde, Hemanth Vamanshankar.

Defects <1 cm in size are usually repaired with avascular grafts, while larger defects >3 cm are repaired by vascularized flaps.[27] The reconstruction plan, however, must be individualized to each patient. Free tissue grafts are easy to harvest with minimum donor site morbidity. However, cases involving high-flow CSF leaks, large dural defects, prior history of surgery or radiation, and benign intracranial hypertension are more prone to graft failure and hence, vascularized flaps are preferred here. Vascularized flaps are more reliable, heal faster than grafts and are for salvage purposes, when locoregional options are unavailable or have failed.[28–30] The nasoseptal flap or Hadad and Bassagaisteguy flap is the workhorse of skull base reconstruction, as it has a wide arc of rotation and can cover defects of the anterior cranial fossa, transsphenoidal and transclival defects independently[31] and can be harvested from either side of the nasal septum, usually the side opposite to the tumor. An endoscopic Doppler probe can be used to verify the artery's presence in the case of a wide sphenoidotomy done previously.[32] What is more important than the size of the defect, is whether the borders of the defect can be identified and exposed. This determines the ease, complexity, or impossibility of the procedure.[33]

High-risk factors which may contribute to a CSF leak prior to reconstruction must be kept in mind. Presence of obesity, prior history of radiation or surgery, and Cushing's disease are considered risk factors. Anterior skull base defects are more common than clival defects. Intraoperatively, high-flow CSF leaks and procedures requiring dissection into ventricles and arachnoid cisterns are associated with higher post-operative leaks.[34]

Small defects are repaired by a simple soft tissue overlay graft. Moderate-sized defects with normal underlying ICPs are reconstructed in a multilayer fashion, using soft tissue for underlay and overlay grafts. Large defects or small defects with elevated ICPs, such as spontaneous CSF leaks or leaks with hydrocephalus, probably benefit from a rigid underlay graft to provide structural support, followed by a soft tissue overlay graft or a vascularized pedicled flap.[20]

Underlay repair is performed by gently elevating the dura above the bony skull base defect and placing grafts in the epidural space. An overlay graft is placed after positioning an appropriate underlay graft. Due care should be taken to prevent iatrogenic mucoceles. An overlay mucosal free graft can be obtained from the nasal septum, middle turbinate, or nasal floor mucosa.

Multiple layers of packing usually follow the overlay graft to give a robust repair. Fat, fascia, and fat followed by gel foam (Pfizer, New York, NY) is usually practiced at our center.

Tissue glues have been extensively used in endoscopic skull base surgery, although their use has been described as "idiosyncratic and typically off-label." Apart from DuraSeal that is approved by FDA as a spine sealant, none of the other tissue glue materials (e.g., Tisseal, Evicel) used are FDA approved for endoscopic skull base surgery.[35] Eloy et al. in their case series have described the use of vascularized septal flaps for high-flow CSF leaks with or without the use of tissue glue. They opine that the use of tissue glues may not provide an added benefit, as suggested by the fact that the only post-operative failure in the study occurred in the sealant group.[36] Complications wise, the possibility of extravasation of tissue glue into intracranial compartment and the inherent property of such materials to swell up after reconstitution (hence, they should not be used in enclosed spaces) should be kept in mind.[37]

Various other techniques for CSF repair have been described such as the bath-plug technique, cufflink, gasket seal method, use of cartilage/bone, obliterative technique, blanket graft technique and the use of human basic fibroblast growth factor (bFGF).[38] The viability of the Hadad flap used in reconstruction of the skull base defects has been assessed by postoperative contrast-enhanced MRI.[39]

Iatrogenic leaks are not that uncommon during endoscopic sinus or skull base surgeries. The leak needs to be addressed and repaired on table if it is identified intraoperatively. The operative video demonstrates an iatrogenic leak during removal of tuberculum sella meningioma and repaired successfully intraoperatively. If the leaks are identified postoperatively, then it should be managed electively as described above (Video 2).

Reconstruction of the skull base defects has been dealt with in detail in Chapter 14.

Nasal pack is usually kept at the end of the surgery. We prefer to keep ivalon (FABCO, New London, CT) or merocel (Medtronic, Jacksonville, FL) nasal packs for 4–5 days under the cover of antibiotics. It is a non-absorbable pack and provides robust support as well as hemostasis. It is removed after removal of the lumbar drain with due care.

## POST-OPERATIVE MANAGEMENT

1. The patient is shifted to an intensive care unit (ICU) and neurologic status is followed closely with regard to the clinical suspicion of intracranial hemorrhage, pneumocephalus, or meningitis.
2. Nasal packs are kept for 4–5 days.
3. Intravenous antibiotics with adequate staphylococcal coverage with blood-brain barrier penetration are continued as long as nasal packs are in place.
4. The patient is placed in a supine position and the lumbar drain is drained at the rate of 10–15 mL/hour for 3–5 days. The drain is then clamped and removed once the patient is stable and there is no evidence of CSF leak.
5. The patient is gradually mobilized and any maneuvers which raise the intracranial pressure like severe coughing, sneezing, or constipation are taken care of.
6. The patient is started on nasal saline spray if there is no evidence of CSF leak for the first month postoperatively.
7. The patient is advised for regular follow up at least once a month for the first 6 months.

## TAKE-HOME POINTS

- Endoscopic management of CSF rhinorrhea is the preferred method of choice in the current scenario.
- Contraindications to endoscopic management are cases in which there are multiple defects of skull base, wide defects, very high-pressure leaks or a very badly deformed skull base.

- The basic principles of reconstruction remain the same; however, there will be some modifications in the technique depending on the site of leak.
- Transpterygoid approach is required for defects involving the lateral recess of the sphenoid sinus.
- The minimal-access combined approach (MACA) is a useful technique in cases involving complicated defects of the frontal sinus.
- Reconstruction of the defect can be done by underlay, overlay or a combined underlay and overlay technique.
- Monopolar cautery should be avoided near or adjacent to the lamina papyracea, optic nerve, or the carotid arteries to avoid complications like blindness or uncontrollable bleeding.
- Grafts, flaps, and adjuvants are used in reconstruction of the defect. Grafts can be autologous, acellular human dermis or engineered collagen. Flaps can be pedicled or free flaps.
- Fluoroscein and navigation are important adjuvants in the management of CSF rhinorrhea.

## VIDEOS

Video 1  MACA – minimal-access combined approach for frontal sinus leak repair.

Video 2  Iatrogenic leak repair – tuberculum sella meningioma.

Video 3  Multiple site CSF leak repair.

Video 4  Ethmoid roof leak repair.

Video 5  Lateral recess of sphenoid leak repair.

## REFERENCES

1. McCudden CR, Senior BA, Hainsworth S, et al. Evaluation of high resolution gel b(2)-transferrin for detection of cerebrospinal fluid leak. *Clin Chem Lab Med* 2013; 51(2): 311–315.
2. Meurman OH, Irjala K, Suonpää J, Laurent B. A new method for the identification of cerebrospinal fluid leakage. *Acta Otolaryngol* 1979; 87(3–4): 366–369.
3. Mathias T, Levy J, Fatakia A, McCoul ED. Contemporary approach to the diagnosis and management of cerebrospinal fluid rhinorrhoea. *Ochsner J* 2016; 16(2): 136–142.
4. Ommaya AK. Spinal fluid fistulae. *Clin Neurosurg* 1976; 23: 363–392
5. Kaufman B, Nulsen FE, Weiss MH, et al. Acquired spontaneous, nontraumatic normal-pressure cerebrospinal fluid fistulas originating from the middle fossa. *Radiology* 1977; 122(2): 379–387.
6. Eljamel MS. Fractures of the middle third of the face and cerebrospinal fluid rhinorrhoea. *Br J Neurosurg* 1994; 8(3): 289–293.

7. Psaltis AJ, Schlosser RJ, Banks CA, Yawn J, Soler ZM. A systematic review of the endoscopic repair of cerebrospinal fluid leaks. *Otolaryngol Head Neck Surg* 2012; 147(2): 196–203.
8. Rangel-Castilla L, Gopinath S, Robertson CS. Management of intracranial hypertension. *Neurol Clin* 2008; 26(2): 521–541.
9. Zweig JL, Carrau RL, Celin SE, et al. Endoscopic repair of cerebrospinal fluid leaks to the sinonasal tract: Predictors of success. *Otolaryngol Head Neck Surg* 2000; 123(3): 195–201.
10. Chaaban MR, Illing E, Riley KO, Woodworth BA. Spontaneous cerebrospinal fluid leak repair: A five-year prospective evaluation. *Laryngoscope* 2014; 124(1): 70–75.
11. McCudden CR, Senior BA, Hainsworth S, et al. Evaluation of high resolution gel b(2)-transferrin for detection of cerebrospinal fluid leak. *Clin Chem Lab Med* 2013; 51(2): 311–315.
12. Thurtell MJ, Wall M. Idiopathic intracranial hypertension (pseudotumor cerebri): Recognition, treatment, and ongoing management. *Curr Treat Options Neurol* 2013; 15(1): 1–12.
13. Martin TJ, Loehrl TA. Endoscopic CSF leak repair. *Curr Opin Otolaryngol Head Neck Surg* 2007; 15(1): 35–39.
14. Bell RB, Dierks EJ, Homer L, Potter BE. Management of cerebrospinal fluid leak associated with craniomaxillofacial trauma. *J Oral Maxillofac Surg* 2004; 62(6): 676–684.
15. Mincy JE. Posttraumatic cerebrospinal fluid fistula of the frontal fossa. *J Trauma* 1966; 6(5): 618–622.
16. Currarino G, Maravilla KR, Salyer KE. Transsphenoidal canal (large craniopharyngeal canal) and its pathologic implications. *Am J Neuroradiol* 1985; 6(1): 39–43.
17. Tomazic PV, Stammberger H. Spontaneous CSF-leaks and meningoencephaloceles in sphenoid sinus by persisting Sternberg's canal. *Rhinology* 2009; 47(4): 369–374.
18. Ecin G, Oner AY, Tokgoz N, et al. T2-weighted vs. intrathecal contrast-enhanced MR cisternography in the evaluation of CSF rhinorrhoea. *Acta Radiol* 2013; 54(6): 698–701.
19. Seth R, Rajasekaran K, Benninger MS, Batra PS. The utility of intrathecal fluorescein in cerebrospinal fluid leak repair. *Otolaryngol Head Neck Surg* 2010; 143(5): 626–632.
20. Schlosser RJ, Bolger WE. Endoscopic management of cerebrospinal fluid rhinorrhoea. *Otolaryngol Clin North Am* 2006; 39(3): 523–538, ix. doi:10.1016/j.otc.2006.01.001.
21. Wolf G, Greistorfer K, Stammberger H. Endoscopic detection of cerebrospinal fluid fistulas with a fluorescence technique: Report of experiences with over 925 cases. *Laryngorhinooto-logie* 1997; 76: 588–594.
22. Bolger WE, Osenbach R. Endoscopic trans pterygoid approach to the lateral sphenoid recess. *Ear Nose Throat J* 1999; 78: 36–46.

23. Karligkiotis A, Pistochini A, Turri-Zanoni M, et al. Endoscopic endonasal orbital transposition to expand the frontal sinus approaches *Am J Rhinol Allergy* 2015; 29(6): 449–456. doi:10.2500/ajra.2015.29.4230.

24. Mantravadi AV, Welch KC. Chapter 26 - Repair of cerebrospinal fluid leak and encephalocele of the cribriform plate. *Atlas of Endoscopic Sinus and Skull Base Surgery* (2nd ed.). In Chiu AG, Palmer JN, Adappa ND (Eds.). Philadelphia, PA: Elsevier, 2019, pp. 223–232.e1

25. Schlosser RJ, Bolger WE. Nasal cerebrospinal fluid leaks: Critical review and surgical considerations. *Laryngoscope* 2004; 114: 255–265.

26. Hoffmann TK, El Hindy N, Müller OM, et al. Vascularised local and free flaps in anterior skull base reconstruction. *Eur Arch Otorhinolaryngol* 2013; 270: 899–907.

27. Zanation AM, Thorp BD, Parmar P, et al. Reconstructive options for endoscopic skull base surgery. *Otolaryngol Clin North Am* 2011; 44(5): 1201–22.

28. Snyderman CH, Kassam AB, Carrau R, et al. Endoscopic reconstruction of cranial base defects following endonasal skull base surgery. *Skull Base* 2007; 17: 73–78.

29. Hegazy HM, Carrau RL, Snyderman CH, et al. Transnasal endoscopic repair of cerebrospinal fluid rhinorrhoea: A meta-analysis. *Laryngoscope* 2000; 110: 1166–1172.

30. Woodworth BA, Prince A, Chiu AG, et al: Spontaneous CSF leaks: A paradigm for definitive repair and management of intracranial hypertension. *Otolaryngol Head Neck Surg* 2008; 138: 715–720.

31. Pinheiro-Neto CD, Prevedello DM, Carrau RL, et al. Improving the design of the pedicled nasoseptal flap for skull base reconstruction: A radioanatomic study. *Laryngoscope* 2007; 117(9): 1560–1569.

32. Pinheiro-Neto CD, Carrau RL, Prevedello DM, et al. Use of acoustic Doppler sonography to ascertain the feasibility of the pedicled nasoseptal flap after prior bilateral sphenoidotomy. *Laryngoscope* 2010; 120: 1798–1801.

33. Turri-Zanoni M, Zocchi J, Lambertoni A, et al. Endoscopic endonasal reconstruction of anterior skull base defects: What factors really affect the outcomes? *World Neurosurg* 2018; 116: e436–e443.

34. Kim GG, Hang AX, Mitchell CA, Zanation AM. Pedicled extranasal flaps in skull base reconstruction. *Adv Otorhinolaryngol* 2013; 74: 71–80.

35. Prickett KK, Wise SK. Grafting materials in skull base reconstruction. *Adv Otorhinolaryngol* 2013; 74: 24–32.

36. Eloy JA, Choudhry OJ, Friedel ME, Kuperan AB, Liu JK. Endoscopic nasoseptal flap repair of skull base defects: As addition of a dural sealant necessary? *Otolaryngol Head Neck Surg* 2012; 147: 161–166.

37. Epstein NE. Dural repair with four spinal sealants: Focused review of the manufacturers' inserts and the current literature. *Spine J* 2010; 10: 1065–1068.

38. Shah NJ. *Chapter 8- Surgical therapy- Step by Step CSF Rhinorrhoea (Endoscopic Nasal Repair).* New Delhi, India: Jaypee Publications, 2009, pp. 42–56.
39. Jyotirmay H, Saxena SK, Ramesh AS, Nagarajan K, Bhat S. Assessing the viability of hadad flap by postoperative contrast-enhanced magnetic resonance imaging. *J Clin Diagn Res* 2017; 11(6): MC01–MC03.

# 10

# Transcranial management of CSF rhinorrhea

HARSH DEORA, NISHANTH SADASHIVA,
MOHAMMED NADEEM

# INTRODUCTION

Cerebrospinal fluid leak through the nose or rhinorrhea is the leakage of a clear watery nutrient-rich fluid that circulates in the brain and spinal cord into the nose. Eighty percent of cerebrospinal fluid (CSF) leaks occur following non-surgical trauma and complicate 2% of all head traumas, and 12% to 30% of all basilar skull fractures. These are associated with morbidities such as general malaise and headache. More importantly, they can lead to potentially life-threatening complications such as meningitis. Thus, they require a thorough and timely evaluation and treatment. CSF leaks occur when the bony cranial vault and its underlying dura are breached. Such leaks may be broadly categorized as traumatic or nontraumatic in origin. Traumatic causes can be further subclassified into surgical and nonsurgical, with surgical causes divided into planned (as in the failure of reconstruction of a planned dural resection) or unplanned (as a complication following an ethmoidectomy or clinoidectomy or paradoxical leak). Nontraumatic CSF leaks may be subclassified into high or normal pressure leaks, with the recognition that tumors can occupy either subclass by mass effect in the high-pressure group, or by the direct erosive effect on the skull base in the normal-pressure group. If no cause can be found, the leak may be classified as idiopathic; however, with careful history taking, physical examination (including nasal endoscopy), and radiologic evaluation, true idiopathic leaks are rare. Endoscope-assisted endonasal cranial base surgery provides an alternative to traditional open approaches. For primarily midline encephaloceles, meningoceles, or CSF leaks, this approach offers the potential for similar defect repair but with a reduced incidence of overall complications. Although otolaryngologists were the first to adopt these techniques to repair CSF leaks, many neurosurgeons have adopted endoscopic techniques, and some leaks still require an open transcranial approach. In this chapter, we are going to look at the open or transcranial route of management of CSF rhinorrhea, including the presentation, diagnosis, and methods of conservative management.

# EPIDEMIOLOGY

Almost 80% of all CSF leaks result from traumatic fractures and its sequelae, 16% from surgical procedures (although this number is rising), and the remaining 4% are nontraumatic. Of the traumatic leaks, more than 50% are evident within the first 2 days, 70% within the first week and almost all present within the first 3 months. The delayed presentation can result from wound contraction or scar formation, necrosis of bony edges or soft tissue, slow resolution of edema, devascularization of tissues or progressive increases in intracranial pressure (secondary to brain edema or other processes). As with most maxillofacial trauma, traumatic CSF leaks occur most commonly in young males and complicate 2% of all head traumas, and 12% to 30% of all basilar skull fractures. Anterior skull base leaks are more common than middle or posterior leaks, due to the firm adherence of the dura to the anterior basilar skull. The most common sites of CSF rhinorrhea following accidental trauma are the sphenoid sinus (30%), frontal sinus (30%), and ethmoid/cribriform (23%). Temporal bone fractures with a resultant CSF leak can present with CSF otorrhea or rhinorrhea via the egress of CSF through the Eustachian tube with an intact tympanic membrane. Although a rare complication of functional endoscopic sinus surgery (FESS), the frequency in which this procedure is performed makes it a significant cause of CSF leaks. When looking at surgical trauma, the most common sites of CSF leak following FESS are ethmoid/cribriform (80%), followed by the frontal sinus (8%) and sphenoid sinus (4%). After neurosurgical procedures, the most common site of CSF leak is the sphenoid sinus (67%) because of the high number of pituitary tumors that are addressed via the transsphenoidal approach.

## CLASSIFICATION

Ommaya proposed dividing CSF rhinorrhea into the classes of traumatic leaks and non-traumatic leaks, and was the first to recognize the importance of accurate classification. In Ommaya's theory that was postulated in 1968, focal atrophy was thought of as a cause of the non-traumatic leak. He suggested that the normal contents of the cribriform plate or sella turcica can become reduced in bulk, possibly because of ischemia. The empty space becomes a pouch filled with CSF. The normal pressure pulse causes this pouch to exert a focal and continually erosive effect, analogous to the creation of the cranial vault excavations, and this can possibly lead to a CSF fistula. However, most authors thought the application of the term "spontaneous" to cases of CSF rhinorrhea was inappropriate because, in their experience, appropriate investigations of all cases of CSF rhinorrhea reveal the true proximate cause. Because most causes of so-called spontaneous rhinorrhea have a specific etiology, the term "spontaneous" is probably best reserved for cases of true idiopathic CSF rhinorrhea in which various investigations cannot determine a specific cause.

In accordance with the theory, CSF rhinorrhoea can be classified as:

1. Traumatic (accidental)
   a. Immediate
   b. Delayed
2. Traumatic (surgical)
   a. Neurosurgical
   b. Oto/rhinological
3. Non-traumatic
   a. Elevated intracranial pressure: neoplasm, hydrocephalus, benign intracranial hypertension
   b. Normal intracranial pressure: congenital anomaly, skull base neoplasms, or erosive processes
4. Idiopathic

## PRESENTATION

Traumatic CSF rhinorrhea cases will usually present with a history suggestive of trauma with a unilateral watery nasal discharge, often associated with a salty taste that occurs on the side of the presumed CSF leak. Most people will report a headache usually made worse by standing, typically becoming prominent throughout the day, with the pain becoming less severe when lying down. Orthostatic headaches can become chronic and disabling to the point of incapacitation. Some patients with spontaneous CSF rhinorrhea will develop headaches that begin in the afternoon. This is known as a "second-half-of-the-day headache." This may be an initial presentation of a spontaneous CSF leak or appear after treatment such as an epidural patch, and likely indicates a slow CSF leak. A low-pressure headache will be caused when the leak allows sufficient CSF to escape in a normal pressure situation. The headache is relieved by reclining or straining, thereby returning the ICP to normal levels. In high-pressure headaches, the pain is relieved by the rhinorrhea. This headache is caused by increased ICP and should alert the clinician to the possibility of concomitant hydrocephalus. Moreover, anosmia may be noted, which suggests a cribriform plate fracture with olfactory tract trauma.

In addition to headache, there can be a feeling of vertigo, facial numbness or weakness, unusually blurry or double vision, neuralgia, fatigue, or a metallic taste in the mouth. Leaking CSF can sometimes be felt or observed as a discharge from the nose or ear. In cases where the leak has been present for a long duration, it may be complicated with episodes of meningitis which will usually present with neck stiffness or fever. Lack of CSF pressure and volume allows the brain to sag and descend through the foramen magnum (large opening) of the occipital bone, at the base of the skull. The lower portion of the brain can stretch or impact one or more cranial nerve complexes, thereby causing a variety of sensory symptoms related to the nerve.

The type of trauma can also be a clue. Fain and colleagues[1] reported an analysis of 80 cases of trauma to the cranial base, and from these determined that there are 5 types of frontonasal trauma:

1. Type I involves only the anterior wall of the frontal sinus.
2. Type II involves the face (a craniofacial disjunction of the Lefort II type or "crush face"), extending upward to the cranial base and to the anterior wall of the frontal sinus, because of the facial retrusion.
3. Type III involves the frontal part of the skull and extends down to the cranial base.
4. Type IV is a combination of types II and III.
5. Type V involves only ethmoid or sphenoid bones.

In this study, CSF leaks were infrequent in types I and II but occurred more frequently in types III, IV, and V, which included a dural tear in each case.

Therefore, when a patient presents with one of these fractures a CSF leak should be suspected.

Although it seems trivial, the final diagnosis of CSF rhinorrhea may be confusing. Other rhinology pathology, including seasonal allergic rhinitis, perennial nonallergic rhinitis, and vasomotor rhinitis, are relatively common, and may mimic some of the signs and symptoms of CSF rhinorrhea or may occur simultaneously with a CSF leak. Furthermore, CSF rhinorrhea is often intermittent, even after trauma, which may lead to false-negative results on diagnostic testing if testing is performed during the quiescent phase. Lastly, the subarachnoid cistern is a relatively low-pressure system. Thus, leaks may be of low volume, which can lead to false-negative testing or failure to recognize that a leak even exists. In cases of high clinical suspicion and initially negative diagnostic testing, further follow-up with repeat testing is warranted.

The presentations of spontaneous CSF rhinorrhea are variable and not very well documented. Obesity is a very important risk factor as it increases intra-abdominal and intrathoracic pressure. This may affect blood circulation in cranial venous collectors and lead to the development of permanent benign intracranial hypertension. Spontaneous CSF leak might also occur secondary to focal atrophy of the olfactory nerve in the region of the cribriform plate. Additionally, defective development of the bony skull base could allow the arachnoid and brain tissue to protrude through the nose. Spontaneous CSF leaks are idiopathic in nature; however, recent evidence has led us to realize that spontaneous CSF rhinorrhea is, in reality, secondary to an intracranial process, namely elevated intracranial pressure (ICP), as well as with factors such as sneezing, coughing, or other causes of normal fluctuations in cerebrospinal fluid pressure.

## INVESTIGATION

### Clinical – halo sign

Traditionally, the presence of a halo sign (the clear ring surrounding a central bloody spot) on gauze, tissue, or linen has been used to predict CSF leak following trauma. This halo forms as blood and CSF separate; however, this test should only be used to arouse suspicion as tears, saliva, and other non-CSF rhinorrhea can give false-positive results. Historically, the components of the rhinorrhea (including glucose, protein, and electrolytes) have been measured to confirm the diagnosis of CSF. These tests, however, should not be relied on, as their sensitivity and specificity are unacceptably low. Detection of glucose in the sample fluid using Glucostix test strips has been a traditional method for the detection of the presence of CSF in nasal and ear discharge. Glucose detection using Glucostix test strips is not recommended as a confirmatory test due to its lack of specificity and sensitivity. Interpretation of the results is confounded by various factors such as contamination from a glucose-containing fluid (tears, nasal mucus, blood in nasal mucus) or relatively low CSF glucose levels.

## Laboratory

Beta-2 transferrin has emerged as a highly sensitive and specific way of identifying CSF, and is now the preferred method of confirming a fluid as CSF. The method was initially discovered in 1979 by Meurman et al.[2] who, when performing protein electrophoresis of CSF, tears, nasal secretions, and serum, noted a β-2 transferrin fraction only in the CSF samples. Techniques for isolating this marker have been subsequently simplified and refined, leading to enhanced sensitivity and specificity. As with any test, a reliable result requires an adequate sample. Of note, although quite specific, there are reports of β-2 transferrin being detected in aqueous humor and in the serum of patients with alcohol-related chronic liver disease. β-2 transferrin is a carbohydrate-free isoform of transferrin, which is almost exclusively found in the CSF. β-2 transferrin is not present in the blood, nasal mucus, tears, or mucosal discharge and does not disturb the test.

Beta-trace protein (βTP) is another marker that has been used for the detection of CSF. This protein is produced by the meninges and choroid plexus and is released into CSF. It is present in other body fluids, including serum, but at much lower concentrations than in CSF. Detection of βTP has 100% sensitivity and specificity in cases of confirmed CSF rhinorrhea, but cannot be reliably used in patients with renal insufficiency or bacterial meningitis, because serum and CSF levels of βTP substantially increase with reduced glomerular filtration rate and decrease with bacterial meningitis.

## Localization

Once a leak has been confirmed, it may be wise to perform a nasal endoscopy in case of doubt, and to confirm findings. However, findings may be non-specific like glistening of the nasal mucosa, but occasionally active leaks can be identified. Eventually, even after direct visualization, imaging of the skull base is critical to localization of CSF leaks, particularly traumatic leaks. Intrathecal agents have been used both to confirm the presence of, and to attempt to, localize CSF leaks. These agents are administered via lumbar puncture into the subarachnoid space and, as such, complications can be severe. Visible dyes, radiopaque dyes, and radioactive markers have been used with a positive result being visualization, either directly or radiographically, of the agent within the nose and paranasal sinuses. Intrathecal fluorescein is the most popular visible agent. Popularized by Messerklinger,[3] intrathecal fluorescein has been associated with multiple complications, including grand mal seizures, and even death. However, in a study of 420 administrations low-dose (50 mg or less) intrathecal fluorescein was found to be useful in localizing CSF fistulas and was deemed unlikely to be associated with adverse events, as most complications were dose-related. The currently recommended dilution is 0.1 mL of 10% intravenous fluorescein (not ophthalmic preparation) in 10 mL of the patient's own CSF, which is infused slowly over 30 minutes. Patients should be extensively counseled about the risks, as this use is not approved by the US Food and Drug Administration.

# RADIOLOGY

## High-resolution CT

High-resolution CT (HRCT) scanning uses 1–2 mm sections in both the coronal and axial planes with a bone algorithm, resulting in localization of the majority of skull base defects that result in CSF leak. However, it is important to recognize that congenital or acquired thinning or absence of portions of the bony skull base may be identified and may not necessarily correspond to the site of CSF leak. However, the real advantage is its use with neuronavigation, and the image guidance it provides. Due to the relative ease of obtaining this study and a high degree of accuracy, this method should be used as the primary imaging modality for traumatic CSF leaks. Plain CT scans may lead to false-positive results secondary to volume averaging, and their use should be limited. The use of intrathecal fluorescein in combination with HRCT allows for the identification of most CSF leaks.

### CT CISTERNOGRAPHY

CT cisternography needs the administration of intrathecal radiopaque contrast (metrizamide, iohexol, or iopamidol) followed by CT scanning. Studies have shown that approximately 80% of CSF leaks can be confirmed through this technology. Weaknesses of this technology include its invasive nature, which can limit its use particularly in the pediatric population, as well as its low sensitivity in intermittent leaks. Positive findings usually reveal pooling of contrast in the frontal or sphenoid sinuses, but may not necessarily locate the actual defect. Furthermore, the density of the dye may obscure bony anatomy, leading to more difficulty in locating the bony defect. Other radioactive markers have been used to detect CSF leaks, including radioactive iodine (131I)-labeled serum albumin, technetium (99mTc)-labeled serum albumin or diethylenetriamine penta-acetic acid (DTPA), and radioactive indium (111In)-labeled DTPA. This technique is similar to intrathecal fluorescein and involves the administration of the tracer via a lumbar puncture. Intranasal pledgets are placed in defined locations under endoscopic guidance and analyzed for tracer uptake approximately 12 to 24 hours later. A scintillation camera is also used but has poor resolution and difficulty precisely localizing the leak.

### MAGNETIC RESONANCE IMAGING

Unlike the above techniques, this is a non-invasive method to diagnose CSF leaks and hence has rapidly gained popularity and acceptance. Here, T2-weighted images with fat suppression and image reversal are used to highlight CSF. The characteristic signal tracking from the intracranial space to the paranasal sinuses represents a CSF leak. The sensitivity of this test is reported to be 85% to 92%, with 100% specificity. MRI and MR cisternography are able to distinguish inflammatory tissue from meningoencephaloceles; however, bony detail is poor. CT and MRI are complementary studies, with CT providing detailed bony anatomy, particularly skull base dehiscence/fractures, and MRI providing soft-tissue detail, including coincident meningoencephaloceles and incidental intracranial pathology. Modern image-guidance software enables the application of CT-MRI fusion for surgical navigation and results in accurately identifying and localizing the site of CSF leakage in 90% of cases.

# TREATMENT

## Conservative

Even when the leak has been diagnosed, initial treatment consists of strict bed rest and elevation of the head at least 30 degrees. In addition, patients should be advised to refrain from coughing, sneezing, nose-blowing, and straining, or Valsalva maneuvers. Stool softeners are recommended, as well as antiemetics to avoid emesis or retching, antitussives to prevent coughing. The resolution of CSF rhinorrhea increases with a higher duration of conservative management. Overall, a resolution with conservative treatment of CSF fistulas involving temporal bone origin is 60%, whereas anterior skull base defects resolve 26.4% of the time with conservative treatment. If conservative management is extended to 7 days, resolution rates improve to 85%, again with leaks of temporal bone origin healing with a significantly higher rate than those of anterior skull base origin.[4] The main reason for this discrepancy may be anatomic differences in the skull base bone and dural structures that are damaged with trauma to these subsites (i.e., the thin bone of the anterior skull base is more likely to cause significant dural lacerations than the thicker temporal bone).

## CSF diversion

An adjunct to the above is temporary CSF diversion, which is most commonly performed with a lumbar drain but occasionally serial lumbar punctures are pursued. Lumbar drains are passive devices yet they require active management, as CSF cell count, protein and glucose measurements, and cultures should be collected frequently to monitor for meningitis, particularly if systemic signs exist. The average drainage rates are around 10 mL per hour. Optimal drainage lowers CSF pressure to decompress the leak; however, if drainage is too high, severe headaches and pneumocephalus may result from the drawing of air through the skull base defect into the cranial vault. There is also the added risk of meningitis. The benefits are that the addition of CSF diversion to conservative measures raises success rates to 70% to 90% with the average duration of drainage being 6.5 days. Another benefit of this treatment is that it can be performed at the bedside if patients are not stable enough to go to the operating room. Lumbar drains can also be used as an adjunctive treatment to increase the success rates following a variety of surgical repairs.

# TRANSCRANIAL REPAIR OF A CSF LEAK

In a recent meta-analysis, when an open repair was compared to endoscopic repair, recurrence occurred in 13/213 cases (6.1%) in 20 studies in the open cohort, at a mean time to recurrence of 34.3 months (range 1 to 36 months). In the endoscopic cohort, recurrence occurred in 31/814 cases (3.8%) in 38 studies, at a mean time to recurrence of 11.7 months (range 0.5 to 30 months). There was no significant difference in the rate of successful repair of CSF leak, meningocele, or encephalocele in the endoscopic cohort compared with the open group and there was no significant difference in the rate of recurrence between the groups. Even so, lumbar drainage was used more frequently in the open cohort compared with the endoscopic cohort (p < 0.001). Complications were significantly lower in the endoscopic group, including meningitis (3.9% versus 1.1%, p=0.034), abscess/wound infection (6.8% versus 0.7%, p < 0.001), and sepsis (3.8% versus 0%, p=0.003). Perioperative mortality was also significantly lower in the endoscopic group (p < 0.001).[5] Despite these reasons, transcranial repair still has a place in CSF rhinorrhea repair as many cases, especially traumatic, may have too many/extensive deficits to be repaired endoscopically, and thus will need transcranial repair. Also, the open approach allows effective repair of large defects, treatment of any associated intracranial lesions, and has the potential for simultaneous repair of both cranial and facial fractures in a single procedure. The more superior the CSF leak lies on the posterior wall, the more difficult it is to treat it endoscopically. The convex shape of the posterior wall of the frontal sinus contributes to this limitation inaccessibility, as well as a narrow frontal sinus with an anteroposterior distance of <1 cm. Other potential limitations of endoscopic surgery include multiple and comminuted traumatic fractures resulting from trauma, especially those extending into the orbital roof, which require a combination of external and endonasal approaches.

## SURGICAL NUANCES

Dandy,[6] in 1926, reported the first successful repair by using a bifrontal craniotomy for access and a fascia lata graft for repair of a CSF leak. With this approach, access to the cribriform plate region and roof of the ethmoid is obtained via a frontal craniotomy. An extended craniotomy and skull base dissection are required to access defects in the sphenoid sinus. After craniotomy, the brain is retracted and the site of the defect is identified. Multiple tissues can be used for repair including fascia lata grafts, muscle plugs, and pedicled galeal or pericranial flaps. Positioning is critical to the complication-free performance of this craniotomy, and extension with the head in a neutral position has been proven to be most beneficial with respect to midline defects. Pins are placed with the single pin right above and behind the pinna, and the two pins on either side of the pinna, or above. Once the incision is marked behind the hairline, local anesthetic is injected at the incision site and injecting generous amounts of saline in the intended flap helps in thickening the pericranial flap and in easy dissection;

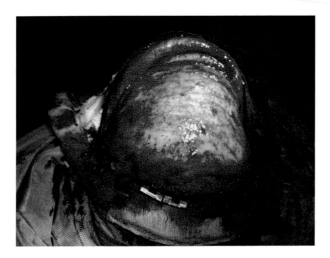

Figure 10.1 Post-skin incision clinical photograph showing incision of the peri-cranial flap. © Harsh Deora, Nishanth Sadashiva, Mohammed Nadeem.

hence, this is useful especially in older individuals, post-traumatic and post-epilepsy cases with dense adhesions (Figure 10.1). Once the incision has been made, it is necessary to be careful not to incise the pericranium, as further graft can be mobilized from the below flap. Elevate the skin flap up to the orbit rim and be mindful of the supra-orbital and supra-trochlear nerve and vessels, avoiding their coagulation while laterally avoiding coagulation of the frontal branch of the superior temporal artery (Figure 10.2). Monopolar electrocautery is then used to disconnect the posterior and lateral attachments of the pericranium (to the superior temporal line) (Figure 10.3). The vascularized graft will be reflected and based anteriorly along the orbital rims (Figure 10.4). The pericranial flap is elevated, stretched, and kept moist during the operation by covering it with a wet piece of sponge. Once the pericranial flap is elevated, ensure the orbital rims are visible, temporalis fascia kept intact for later possible use, and minimum muscle dissection of the key burr hole area only is done.

The usual boundaries of craniotomy are:

- Lower edge: orbital roof
- Upper edge: just anterior to the coronal suture
- Lateral edge: superior temporal line

A smaller variation is sometimes shown with an advance of a smaller bony defect, but leads to unsightly bone cut lines on the forehead and is thus not recommended. In numerous studies, complications due to the bicoronal approach, such as anesthesia or paresthesia of the scalp, wide, and irregular incision scars, temporary or permanent alopecia, were frequently reported; however, a correct flap harvesting with cold scalpel through a subfollicular plane, without

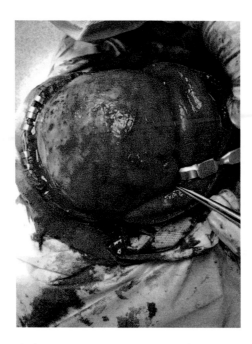

Figure 10.2 Clinical photograph showing extent of the skin flap elevation up to the orbital rim. © Harsh Deora, Nishanth Sadashiva, Mohammed Nadeem.

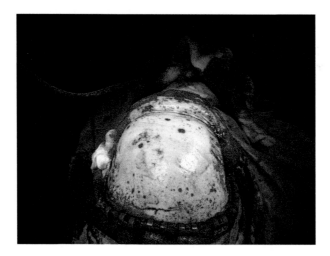

Figure 10.3 Clinical photograph showing boundaries of exposure of the craniotomy post elevation of the pericranial flap. © Harsh Deora, Nishanth Sadashiva, Mohammed Nadeem.

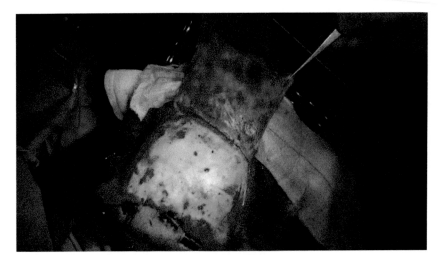

Figure 10.4 Clinical photograph showing vascularized pericranial flap. © Harsh Deora, Nishanth Sadashiva, Mohammed Nadeem.

crossing the supraorbital nerve's plane, allows us to avoid any such kind of these complications.

## FRONTAL SINUS

While traditional teaching has been for the cranialization of the frontal sinus with obliteration (Figures 10.5, 10.6) of the drainage pathway, the current methods of instruction are different. Cranialization was indicated in the setting of fragments insufficient to repair the frontal sinus drainage pathway and low probability of

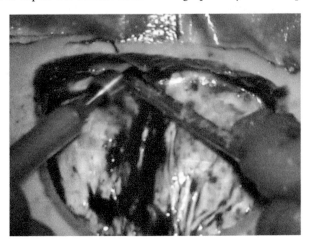

Figure 10.5 Clinical photograph showing post craniotomy cranialization of the frontal sinus. © Harsh Deora, Nishanth Sadashiva, Mohammed Nadeem.

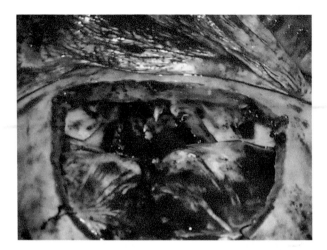

Figure 10.6 Clinical photograph showing obliteration of the frontal sinus using bone wax. © Harsh Deora, Nishanth Sadashiva, Mohammed Nadeem.

postoperative frontal patency. In addition, restoration of the frontal sinus drainage pathway aims at restoring sinus physiologic function and thus avoids frontal sinus obliteration, whenever feasible. In this method, after satisfactory repair had been performed, frontal sinus drainage was inspected for any signs of obstruction or disruption with an angled scope and a rolled silastic sheet was placed in the frontal recess and left in place for three weeks to aid in healing. In all patients, fibrin glue and Surgicel (Ethicon Sàrl, Neuchâtel, Switzerland) were used to tack the overlay graft or flap into position. The nasal cavities are packed with sterile polyvinyl sponges (Merocel; Merocel Surgical Products Corp, Mystic, CT) that are removed 2 days after surgery.[7]

## INTRADURAL STEPS

Once the dura is opened on either side of the sagittal sinus, the same is obliterated and cut using 2 proline/vicryl sutures (Ethicon Sàrl, Neuchâtel, Switzerland) and the dural flap is elevated posteriorly. Any herniated dural or brain tissue (Figure 10.7) was reduced using bipolar electrocautery or coblation (Figure 10.8). It is imperative that at least one of the two olfactory nerves be preserved to prevent loss of sense of smell and taste for an individual (Figure 10.9). A rim of mucosa around the defect edge was removed to prevent mucus production underneath the graft from detaching it, and bony edges were regularized by drilling. In spontaneous CSF leak, benign intracranial hypertension (BIH), or meningocele, the bone around the leak site is often very thin and must be handled cautiously to avoid accidental enlargement of the bone defect. Gentle pressure on the dura mater with a cottonoid pledget creates an epidural space for a graft. Tissue sealants, such as fibrin glue, can be used to hold the graft in position (Figure 10.10); however, this will only last a few weeks, leading the authors to prefer suture closure to the dura distal to the defect (Figure 10.11), which holds the graft more

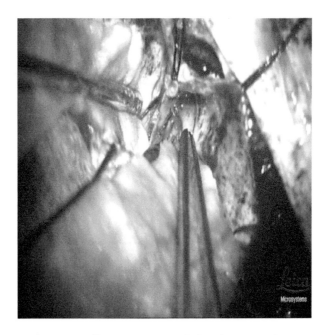

Figure 10.7 Delineation of herniated encephalocele. © Harsh Deora, Nishanth Sadashiva, Mohammed Nadeem.

securely in place. Reported success rates vary; however, recurrence rates as high as 27% have been reported.[8] A clear advantage of this approach is that it provides direct access to the defect and allows for repair of multiple sites; however, with high reported failure rates, the morbidity of a craniotomy, and brain retraction (including potential hematoma, seizures, and anosmia), extracranial techniques

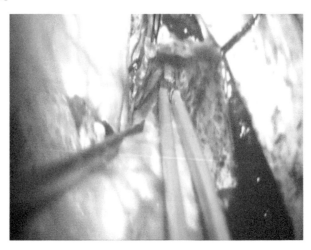

Figure 10.8 Bipolar cautery and release of herniated gliotic brain. © Harsh Deora, Nishanth Sadashiva, Mohammed Nadeem.

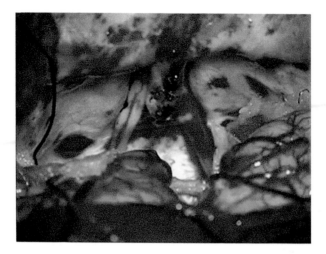

Figure 10.9 Clinical photograph showing olfactory nerves bilaterally preserved after elevation of the dura and brain retraction. © Harsh Deora, Nishanth Sadashiva, Mohammed Nadeem.

are now preferred in most circumstances. At present, these techniques are mostly used in patients who require a craniotomy and exposure of the skull base to treat associated intracranial pathology.

## COMPLICATIONS AND CONTROVERSIES

Bacterial meningitis is the major cause of morbidity and mortality in patients with CSF leaks, making antibiotic prophylaxis a reasonable suggestion and the reported

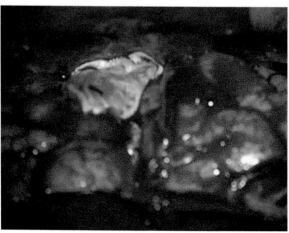

Figure 10.10 Clinical photograph showing vascularized pericranial graft being placed on the anterior cranial fossa base. © Harsh Deora, Nishanth Sadashiva, Mohammed Nadeem.

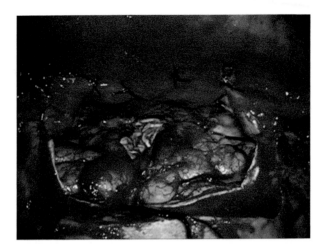

Figure 10.11 Clinical photograph showing flap being sutured on the sphenoid ridge. © Harsh Deora, Nishanth Sadashiva, Mohammed Nadeem.

rates amount to 10% in many series.[5] A Cochrane Database review was performed to address the controversy regarding antibiotic use in these cases.[9] The analysis included 208 patients from 4 randomized controlled trials and an additional 2168 patients from 17 nonrandomized controlled trials. The analysis concluded that the evidence does not support the use of prophylactic antibiotics to reduce the risk of meningitis in patients with basilar skull fractures or basilar skull fractures with active CSF leaks. However, in certain circumstances (such as active bacterial rhinosinusitis or grossly contaminated tract leading to the intracranial cavity), antibiotic coverage is reasonable. Patients with traumatic CSF leaks lasting more than 7 days have been shown to have an estimated eightfold to tenfold increase in the risk of meningitis.[10–12] Harvey and colleagues[13] looked to address this long-term risk and found that surgical repair results in a decreased incidence of intracranial complications (including meningitis) over the long term. After assessment of risk factors for the development of complications, they concluded that in patients with small nonleaking encephaloceles without adjacent infection, early surgical repair may not be indicated. In traumatic cases, if the defect is in the anterior skull base, conservative treatment should be performed for 3 days. At this point, if the leak persists, consideration of CSF diversion or endoscopic repair should be discussed in a multidisciplinary fashion. If CSF diversion is initiated and the leak is persistent, definitive repair (preferably endoscopic) should be performed around CSF leak day 7. If the CSF leak originates in the temporal bone, conservative measures should be continued for 5 to 7 days, followed by CSF diversion for an additional 7 days, as these are more likely to close spontaneously and less likely to result in meningitis. Further operative repair of these defects cannot be addressed endoscopically, and definitive surgical repair of these defects can carry significant morbidity. If the leak persists for 2 weeks, definitive surgical repair should be performed. Intraoperative CSF leaks recognized at the time of surgery (either FESS or skull base procedures)

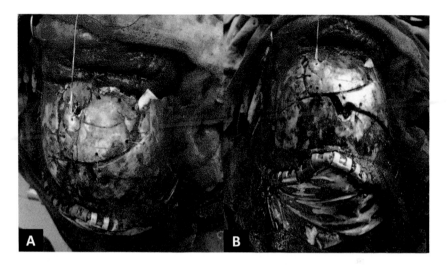

Figure 10.12 Clinical photograph showing the extent of bone defects seen after trauma. (A) Before repair. (B) After repair. © Harsh Deora, Nishanth Sadashiva, Mohammed Nadeem.

should be immediately repaired. For planned dural resections, reconstruction should be "watertight." If recognition is delayed by days, weeks, or months, it is reasonable, although not the authors' practice, to initiate a short period of conservative therapy (a few days to 1 week). The leak should be confirmed and identified and repaired if the leak persists for 1 week, despite conservative measures. One should recognize that the later the CSF leak presents following the procedure, the less likely it is to resolve with conservative measures alone. Moreover, if the leak is massive in nature, early surgical intervention is indicated. In addition to the usual complications of bleeding and surgical site infections, other complications like tension pneumocephalus, meningoencephaloceles, brain abscesses and unsightly defects (Figure 10.12) can also occur, and active investigation with early intervention must be sought in such cases.

## REFERENCES

1. Fain J, Chabannes J, Peri G, et al. Frontobasal injuries and CSF fistulas. Attempt at an anatomy clinical classification. Therapeutic incidence. Neurochirurgie 1975;21(6):493–506 [in French].
2. Meurman OH, Irjala K, Suonpaa J, et al. A new method for the identification of cerebrospinal fluid leakage. Acta Otolaryngol 1979;87:366–9.
3. Messerklinger W. Nasal endoscopy: Demonstration, localization and differential diagnosis of nasal liquorrhea. HNO 1972;20:268–70 [in German].
4. Keerl R, Weber RK, Draf W, et al. Use of sodium fluorescein solution for detection of cerebrospinal fluid fistulas: An analysis of 420 administrations and reported complications in Europe and the United States. Laryngoscope 2004;114:266–72.

5. Komotar RJ, Starke RM, Raper DM, Anand VK, Schwartz TH. Endoscopic endonasal versus open repair of anterior skull base CSF leak, meningocele, and encephalocele: A systematic review of outcomes. *J Neurol Surg A Cent Eur Neurosurg* 2013;74(4):239–50.
6. Dandy WD. Pneumocephalus (intracranial pneumocele or aerocele). *Arch Surg* 1926;12:949–82.
7. Rohrich RJ, Hollier LH. Management of frontal sinus fractures. Changing concepts. *Clin Plast Surg* 1992;19:219–23.
8. Jones V, Virgin F, Riley K, et al. Changing paradigms in frontal sinus cerebrospinal fluid leak repair. *Int Forum Allergy Rhinol* 2012;2:227–32.
9. Ratilal BO, Costa J, Sampaio C. Antibiotic prophylaxis for preventing meningitis in patients with basilar skull fractures. *Cochrane Database Syst Rev* 2006;(1):CD004884.
10. Daudia A, Biswas D, Jones NS. Risk of meningitis with cerebrospinal fluid rhinorrhea. *Ann Otol Rhinol Laryngol* 2007;116(12):902–5.
11. Bernal-Sprekelsen M, Bleda-Vázquez C, Carrau RL. Ascending meningitis secondary to traumatic cerebrospinal fluid leaks. *Am J Rhinol* 2000;14:257–9.
12. Bernal-Sprekelsen M, Alobid I, Mullol J, et al. Closure of cerebrospinal fluid leaks prevents ascending bacterial meningitis. *Rhinology* 2005;43:277–81.
13. Harvey RJ, Smith JE, Wise SK, et al. Intracranial complications before and after endoscopic skull base reconstruction. *Am J Rhinol* 2008;22:516–21.

# 11

# Role of navigation in CSF rhinorrhea

## HEMANTH VAMANSHANKAR AND JYOTIRMAY S HEGDE

Stereotaxis is the principle behind image-guided neuronavigation. The brain can be divided into three imaginary intersecting spatial planes (frontal, horizontal, and sagittal), based on the Cartesian coordinate system. The distance of any specific point within the brain can be measured with reference to these three intersecting planes. By combining such coordinate referencing of the brain with a parallel 3-D image coordinate system, neuronavigation can provide accurate surgical guidance.[1,2] Functional imaging technology like functional magnetic resonance imaging (f-MRI), positron emission tomography (PET), and magnetoencephalography (MEG) have permitted surgical access to almost every area of the brain, with minimal morbidity. Furthermore, the use of intraoperative MRI can document residual lesions and assess brain shift during surgery.[3–12]

The concept of frameless stereotaxy or neuronavigation was developed by Roberts et al. in 1986. This was based on an ultrasound emitting source and microphone attached to the microscope, the data of which was processed by a computer.[13] Navigation based on magnetic sources, and which was frameless and armless, was developed by Kato et al. in 1991.[14] Zamorano et al. developed a device for navigation based on optoelectronic measuring principles using infrared LEDs as emitting sources, in 1993.[15] A navigation arm with six degrees of freedom and high precision potentiometers was developed in 1993 by Koivukangas.[16] The first landmark neurosurgical procedure using navigation was performed in 1995, using a 0.5T iMR imaging suite (also known as the General Electric "double doughnut") containing a 56 cm-wide gap in the center of the magnet for performing the surgical procedure.[17] An i-CT scanner fixed to an LED-based navigation system was developed by Matula et al. in 1998.[18] Functional neuro-navigation, by fusing MEG data with f-MRI to get 3D images, was developed by Nimsky et al. in 1999. The 3-D images could then be transferred to the navigation microscope.[4] Robot-assisted neuronavigated neuroendoscopy was described in three patients by Zimmermann et al. in 2002.[19] An ultrasonography-based navigation system integrating f-MR and DT imaging data was developed by Rasmussen et al. in 2007.[20]

## STEPS OF NAVIGATION

For the purpose of linking pre- and intraoperative images to the surgical procedure, the following steps are proposed:

- Obtaining pre-operative images: this is in the form of PET, SPECT, fMRI, and magnetoencephalography. The images of various imaging modalities are then fused together to obtain better anatomical resolution in a procedure called "image fusion".
- Patient registration: done by placing fiducial skin markers over the patient's head regions. A minimum of 6, to an optimal of 12–15 markers are placed at different levels to gain better accuracy.
- Localization: A 3D-digitizer is used to recognize emitted or reflected signals produced from the intraoperative instrument. The localization system consists of an optic digitizer camera, reference frame, and the surgical instrument. LED-equipped accessory tools are placed at fixed distances from each other, and attached to the surgical instrument. These emit or reflect light during the surgical procedure.
- Intraoperative control.
- Fusing intraoperative images with pre-operative ones.
- Visualization and surgery[21]

Navigation increases the safety in endoscopic surgery by providing millimetric accuracy of the site of lesion. This in turn helps in performing lesser invasive endoscopic explorations and better chances of closure in CSF leaks. Navigation is particularly useful in cases of trauma or previous surgery, wherein normal anatomical landmarks such as fovea ethmoidalis and middle turbinate are lost.[22] Navigation reduces the length of surgery, shortens the stay at hospital, and reduces the incidence of wound infections.[23]

Contrary to most studies, Taubee et al., in their retrospective review of 24 patients, say that navigation did not improve the success rates of leak closure, although it may improve surgeon confidence.[24] Time-consuming calculations and registration, restriction of view and space in the operating field, are some concerns of present navigation systems.[25,26]

Zhang et al. have proposed the use of a variant of a T2-weighted turbo spin echo sequence called 3D-SPACE (three-dimensional sampling perfection with application-optimized contrast using different flip angle evolution) for navigation. This technique offers high-resolution images (better than conventional T2 imaging) in a 3-D thin slice, without requiring radiation exposure or intrathecal contrast administration. Apart from its use in navigation, it can also provide information as to whether CSF rhinorrhoea exists, its location of leakage (accuracy of up to 1 mm or less), estimate anatomical structures (especially the anterior and lateral wall of sphenoid sinus), and prevent damage to vital neurovascular structures. As compared to a conventional T2W sequence, a 3D-SPACE sequence in detecting a CSF leak had better sensitivity (69.0% Vs 93.1%); specificity (81.3% Vs 87.5%); positive predictive value (87.0% Vs 93.1%); and negative predictive value (59.1% Vs 87.5%).[22]

The usefulness of MRI for detecting CSF leaks and navigation has been described in various studies in the form of intrathecal contrast medium-enhanced magnetic resonance cisternography (CEMRC), T2-weighted MR cisternography and three-dimensional constructive interference in a steady state (3D-CISS).[27–29] Algin et al. report 3D-CISS as a non-invasive and reliable method of CSF leak detection with sensitivity of 76%.[30] Sensitivity and specificity of CEMRC have been reported to range between 80–100% and 53–100% respectively.[27–29]

The future of neuronavigation seems promising. The development of i-CT technology has provided better image quality with no radiation burden, as compared to previous intraoperative CT. Production of MR imaging compatible instruments, and combining i-CR and i-MR imaging, would bring about better imaging quality intra-op. Imaging with SPECT and PET, which is presently not possible in the operating room due to radiation hazards and cost concerns, would open a door of new possibilities.[31] Another exciting field is microscanning, i.e., ultrasonographic scanning at higher frequencies, which can bring about imaging histological specimens in 3-D without the need for staining/sectioning. Wells et al. also describe this technique in gene transfection by delivering high-intensity localized ultrasound to individually targeted cells.[32] Finally, the advent of robotics combined with navigation may enable performing skull base procedures at distant locations with the use of telerobotic technology.

## REFERENCES

1. Golfinos JG, Fitzpatrick BC, Smith LR et al. Clinical use of a frameless stereotactic arm: Results of 325 cases. *J Neurosurg* 1995; 83: 197–205.
2. Selesnick SH, Kackar A. Image guided surgical navigation in otology and neurootology. *Am J Otol* 1999; 20: 688–697.
3. Ganslandt O, Fahlbusch R, Nimsky C et al. Functional neuronavigation with magnetoencephalography: Outcome in 50 patients with lesions around the motor cortex. *J Neurosurg* 1999; 91: 73–79.
4. Nimsky C, Ganslandt O, Kober H et al. Integration of functional magnetic resonance imaging supported by magnetoencephalography in functional neuronavigation. *Neurosurgery* 1999; 44: 1249–1256.

5. Kamada K, Takeuchi F, Kuriki S et al. Functional neurosurgical stimulation with brain surface magnetic resononce imaging and magnetoencephalography. *Neurosurgery* 1993; 33: 269–273.
6. Nimsky C, Ganslandt O, Fahlbusch R et al. Intraoperative use of the Magnetom Open in neurosurgery. *Electromedica* 1999; 67: 2–8.
7. Nimsky C, Ganslandt O, Cerny S et al. Quantification of, visualization of, and compensation for brain shift using intraoperative magnetic resonance imaging. *Neurosurgery* 2000; 47: 1070–1080.
8. Nimsky C, Ganslandt O, Kober H et al. Intraoperative magnetic resonance imaging combined with neuronavigation: A new concept. *Neurosurgery* 2001; 48: 1082–1091.
9. Black P McL, Moriarty T, Alexander E III et al. The development and implementation of intraoperative magnetic resonance imaging and its neurosurgical applications. *Neurosurgery* 1997; 41: 831–845.
10. Black P McL, Alexander E III, Martin C et al. Craniotomy for tumor treatment in an intraoperative magnetic resonance imaging unit. *Neurosurgery* 1999; 45: 423–433.
11. Nabavi A, Black PM, Gering DL et al. Serial intraoperative magnetic resonance imaging of brain shift. *Neurosurgery* 2001; 48: 787–798.
12. Tronnier V, Wirtz C, Knauth M et al. Intraoperative diagnostic and interventional magnetic resonance imaging in neurosurgery. *Neurosurgery* 1997; 40: 891–902.
13. Roberts DW, Strohbehn JW, Hatch JF, Murray W, Kettenberger H. A frameless stereotaxic integration of computerized tomographic imaging and the operating microscope. *J Neurosurg* 1986; 65: 545–549.
14. Kato A, Yoshimine T, Hayakawa T et al. A frameless, armless navigational system for computer-assisted neurosurgery. Technical note. *J Neurosurg* 1991; 74: 845–849.
15. Zamorano LJ, Nolte LP, Kadi AM. Interactive intraoperative localization using infrared-based system. *Neurol Res* 1993; 15: 290–298.
16. Koivukangas J, Louhisalmi Y, Alakuijala J, Oikarinen J. Ultrasound- controlled neuronavigator-guided brain surgery. *J Neurosurg* 1993; 79: 36–42.
17. Black PM, Moriarty T, Alexander EA et al. Development and implementation of intraoperative magnetic resonance imaging and its neurosurgical applications. *Neurosurgery* 1997; 41: 831–845.
18. Matula C, Rössler K, Reddy M, Schindler E, Koos WT. Intraoperative computed tomography guided neuronavigation: Concepts, efficiency, and work flow. *Comput Aided Surg* 1998; 3: 174–182.
19. Zimmermann M, Krishnan R, Raabe A, Seifert V. Robotassisted navigated neuroendoscopy. *Neurosurgery* 2002; 51: 1446–1451.

20. Rasmussen IA Jr, Lindseth F, Rygh OM et al. Functional neuronavigation combined with intra-operative 3D ultrasound: Initial experiences during surgical resections close to eloquent brain areas and future directions in automatic brain shift compensation of preoperative data. *Acta Neurochir* 2007; 149: 365–378.
21. Ivanov M, Ciurea AV. Neuronavigation. Principles. Surgical technique. *J Med Life* 2009; 2(1): 29–35.
22. Zhang Y, Wang F, Chen X et al. Cerebrospinal fluid rhinorrhea: Evaluation with 3D-SPACE sequence and management with navigation-assisted endonasal endoscopic surgery. *Br J Neurosurg* 2016; 30: 643–648. doi: 10.1080/02688697.2016.1199787
23. Wirtz CR, Tronnier VM, Bonsanto MM et al. Neuronavigation. Methods and prospects. *Nervenarzt* 1998; 69: 1029–1036.
24. Tabaee A, Kassenoff TL, Kacker A, Anand VK. The efficacy of computer assisted surgery in the endoscopic management of cerebrospinal fluid rhinorrhea. *Otolaryngol Head Neck Surg* 2005; 133: 936–943.
25. Leksell L. The stereotaxic method and radiosurgery of the brain. *Acta Chir Scand* 1951; 102: 316–319.
26. Archip N, Clatz O, Whalen S et al. Non-rigid alignment of pre-operative MRI, fMRI, and DT-MRI with intra-operative MRI for enhanced visualization and navigation in image-guided neurosurgery. *Neuroimage* 2007; 35: 609–624.
27. Jayakumar PN, Kovoor JM, Srikanth SG, Praharaj SS. 3D steady-state MR cisternography in CSF rhinorrhoea. *Acta Radiol* 2001; 42: 582–584.
28. Selcuk H, Albayram S, Ozer H et al. Intrathecal gadolinium-enhanced MR cisternography in the evaluation of CSF leakage. *Am J Neuroradiol* 2010; 31: 71–75.
29. Arbelaez A, Medina E, Rodriguez M et al. Intrathecal administration of gadopentetate dimeglumine for MR cisternography of nasoethmoidal CSF fistula. *Am J Roentgenol* 2007; 188: W560–W564.
30. Algin O, Hakyemez B, Gokalp G et al. The contribution of 3D-CISS and contrast-enhanced MR cisternography in detecting cerebrospinal fluid leak in patients with rhinorrhoea. *Br J Radiol* 2010; 83:225–232.
31. Enchev Y. Neuronavigation: Geneology, reality, and prospects. *Neurosurg Focus.* 2009; 27(3): E11.
32. Wells PN. Advances in ultrasound: From microscanning to telerobotics. *Br J Radiol* 2000; 73: 1138–1147.

# 12

# Role of radiodiagnosis in CSF rhinorrhea

SHRESHTA BHAT

Cerebrospinal fluid (CSF) leak occurs when there is an osseous and dural defect at the skull base, with direct communication of the subarachnoid space to the extracranial space, usually a paranasal sinus.[1] When the CSF leak is through the nose or paranasal sinuses, it is called CSF rhinorrhea. Its accurate diagnosis is necessary prior to any potential intervention.

The most common site of a CSF fistula is the cribriform plate, followed by the junction of the cribriform plate, and the fovea ethmoidalis.

Cerebrospinal fluid (CSF) rhinorrhea is a potentially dangerous problem. Imaging plays a pivotal role in the early diagnosis of CSF leaks to prevent life-threatening complications such as brain abscess and meningitis.

## IMAGING MODALITIES AND THEIR USES

3-D, isotropic, high-resolution computed tomography (HRCT) accurately detects the site and size of the bony defect. In the case of single and multiple bony defects, CT cisternography helps accurately identify the site of the CSF leak. CSF leaks and associated complications, such as the encephaloceles and meningoceles, are accurately detected and localized by magnetic resonance imaging (MRI) and 3-D

Table 12.1 The imaging modalities for CSF rhinorrhea, their uses and limitations are shown briefly

| Imaging modality | Uses | Limitations |
|---|---|---|
| Radionuclide Cisternography | Intermittent leaks are accurately detected | Radiation, time consuming procedure. |
| HRCT | Localisation and measurement of bony defect | Difficult to differentiate from mucosal pathology |
| 3D T2 DRIVE MR Cisternography | Non-invasive localisation of the leak site | Bony defect is not directly visualised |
| CT Cisternography | Confirmation of location-more effective | Invasive, Radiation |

*HRCT:* high resolution computed tomography, CT: computed tomography, MR: Magnetic resonance imaging.

T2 DRIVE MR cisternography. Radionuclide cisternography can detect occult CSF leaks (Table 12.1).

## HIGH-RESOLUTION COMPUTED TOMOGRAPHY (HRCT)

HRCT of the skull base can accurately detect the site of CSF fistula and classify a dural or osseous defect. It has become a mainstay of the initial screening examination in the diagnosis of a CSF leak. It is reported to have a sensitivity as high as 92% and specificity of 100%.[2] A bone algorithm should always be applied.

Axial images are acquired for the evaluation of the posterior and lateral walls of the sphenoid sinus, the posterior wall of the frontal sinus (Fig. 12.1), and the mastoid complex. Coronal images are acquired for the evaluation of the roof of the ethmoid and sphenoid sinuses, cribriform plates, and tegmen tympani.[3] Volumetric acquisition with multidetector CT imaging and thin collimation allows an isotropic multi-planar reconstruction for the accurate identification of the site of the CSF leak.

The clinching point in diagnosis of the CSF leak is the bone defect with fluid opacification (Fig. 12.2) of adjacent sinuses or an air-fluid level. The dural defect may not be identified. In the evaluation of the temporal bone, a tegmen defect or fracture through an inner ear structure with a unilaterally opacified mastoid and middle ear, indicates a CSF fistula. CT may show a tumor intracranially or of the skull base or meningocele and/or meningoencephalocele, which requires further evaluation with MRI imaging, because in such conditions, the herniating structure is also to be resected along with overlay and underlay repair of the dural defect.

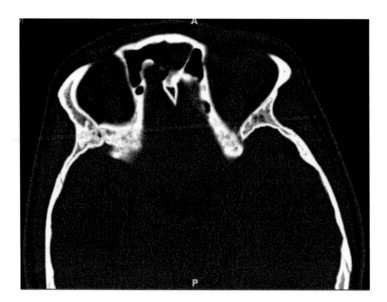

Figure 12.1 Axial images are acquired for evaluation of the posterior wall of the frontal sinus, showing a small defect with soft tissue density adjacent to it. © Shreshta Bhat.

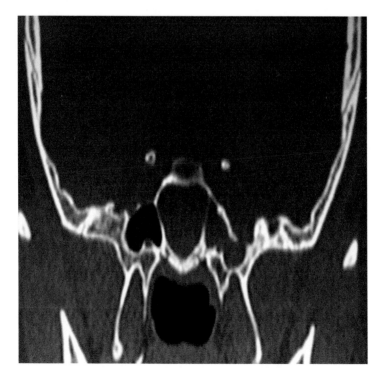

Figure 12.2 Coronal CT demonstrating the most common site of CSF fistula, i.e., the cribriform plate. © Shreshta Bhat.

The CT data also provides intraoperative image guidance for the endoscopic repair of a CSF leak.

An evaluation of the temporal bone along with anterior skull base is recommended in cases of temporal bone trauma when an occult CSF otorrhea with intact tympanic membrane presents with CSF rhinorrhea.

Shetty et al.,[4] in their evaluation of the role of HRCT and MR cisternography in the diagnosis of CSF leaks, identified that the thinner sections that are possible with HRCT yielded better results when compared to MR examination. MR cisternography's accuracy, sensitivity, and specificity were 89%, 87%, and 100% respectively as opposed to HRCT, which showed an accuracy of 92%, sensitivity of 92% and specificity of 100%. When multiple bony defects are seen on HRCT, it is difficult to identify the defect that is primarily responsible for the CSF leak, hence by superimposing the CT and MR data, we can accurately localize the CSF leaks with a sensitivity of 89%.[5]

Limitations: Partial volume averaging can cause both false-negative and false-positive findings. Inaccuracies can be minimized by using the thinnest sections possible but at the expense of a significantly higher radiation dose to the eye.

## CT CISTERNOGRAPHY

CT cisternography is the examination of choice for the evaluation of an active CSF leak. A non-contrast HRCT of the skull base in the axial plane is combined with CT cisternography for the precise anatomical localization of the osseous defect and definitive proof of the CSF leak. In addition, nasal pledgets can be placed prior to CT cisternography to confirm the presence of the CSF leak on imaging.

An intrathecal injection of approximately 3–10 mL, of an iodinated non-ionic low-osmolar contrast agent, is performed. The patient is positioned in a Trendelenburg position to opacify the basal cisterns or prone, with the head in the dependent position, followed by CT imaging immediately with a thin section coronal CT scan of the skull base done (maxillofacial or temporal region). A positive result involves the presence of a skull base defect (Fig. 12.3) and contrast opacification (Fig. 12.4) within the sinus, nasal cavity, or middle ear; or an increase in Hounsfield units of greater than 50%, after CT cisternography.[6] The acquisition of pre-cisternography images is important to differentiate extracranial contrast material accumulation from benign high-attenuation inspissated sinus secretions, sclerotic sinus walls, or blood. For accurate results, optimal window level settings are chosen on the workstation.

After the administration of a contrast agent, elevating the intracranial pressure reportedly yields better results; however, due to potential complications of severe headache or widening the defect, we do not perform this technique.[7]

Advantages: especially performed for patients with multiple skull base fractures and/or defects, patients with negative CT scans, or those in whom the diagnosis is in question. The overall sensitivity of CT cisternography is 92% in active leaks, 40% in inactive leaks[8] and only 48% in cases with intermittent leaks.[6]

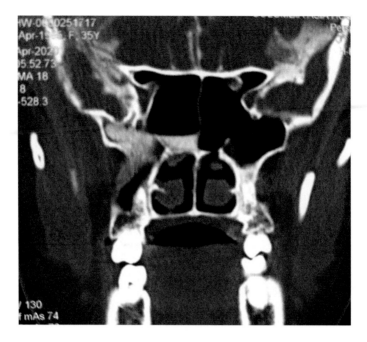

Figure 12.3  CT cisternography with extravasation of the contrast agent through a right lateral recess of the sphenoid bone defect. © Shreshta Bhat.

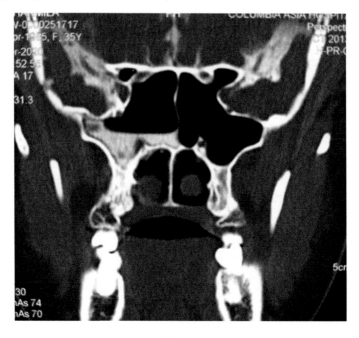

Figure 12.4  CT cisternography with fluid level of the contrast agent within the right sphenoid sinus. © Shreshta Bhat.

Limitations: CT cisternography is a minimally invasive procedure, but the limitations are headache, meningeal irritation, and rarely, seizures. The headache and meningeal irritation are relatively common and are seen in approximately 10% of patients undergoing CT cisternography.[1]

A small but inherent risk of infection and lumbar CSF leak is present. A very low incidence of the major side effects seen include headache, meningeal irritation, and seizures. Any invasive cisternography is relatively contraindicated in patients with meningitis or elevated intracranial pressure.

The two examinations, CT-cisternography and radionuclide cisternography, can be combined in the most complex cases, when the presence of a leak is questionable and after all other imaging findings have been unrevealing. But we find this approach is not cost-effective.

## MR CISTERNOGRAPHY

MR cisternography is one of the robust techniques for the demonstration of CSF leaks and can assess possible encephalocele or meningoencephalocele (Fig. 12.5). The MR cisternography studies are performed on 1.5 Tesla and high-strength MRI scanners. The principle of MR cisternography is to demonstrate a contiguous fluid signal between the cisternal space and nasal sinus on heavily weighted T2 images (Fig. 12.6).

Position: One of the basic principles of imaging CSF fistula is to keep the patient in the prone position which will provoke the leak. For patients who are not comfortable in laying prone for long time, a supine position can also be used.

A complete study of MR cisternography takes approximately 20 min. Initially, T2W axial sections of the brain and skull base are obtained to rule out intracranial mass lesions. The identification of the exact site of the CSF leak depends on

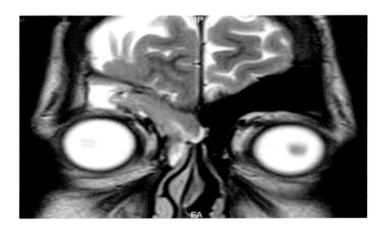

Figure 12.5 T2-weighted MRI, showing a right frontal roof defect with encephalo-meningocele appearing as neuroparenchyma within the right frontal sinus. © Shreshta Bhat.

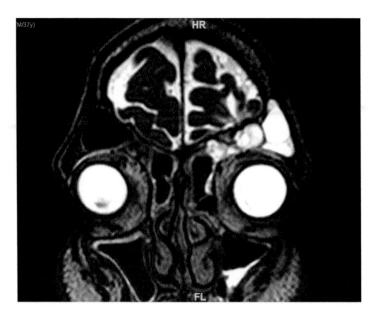

Figure 12.6 Heavily T2-weighted gradient sequence, MRI, showing a frontal left lateral defect with fluid intensity within, suggesting an active CSF leak. © Shreshta Bhat.

the acquisition of images on heavily T2W sequences to enhance conspicuousness of the fistulous tract and gradient sequences such as 3-D T2 DRIVE (driven-equilibrium pulse sequence), CISS (Siemens), B FFE (Philips), FIESTA (GE) on a 1.5 T or higher scanner.

Sequences in detail:

- Thin 1–1.5 mm coronal sections, using a 3-D T2 DRIVE sequence, which in turn uses 3-D turbo-spin echo (TSE) technique for producing high-resolution T2-weighted images. It has low sensitivity for flow voids but high signal-to-noise ratio.
- A DRIVE pulse uses 90° radiofrequency pulse with gradient refocusing pulse and a spoiled gradient. This 90° pulse is given exactly when the echo appears to rebuild the vertical magnetization in the fluid.
  - To achieve a short scan time, the TSE factor should be set to the highest possible value, and a short TR is used.
  - Contiguous interleaved images are obtained at a slice thickness of 2 mm and a field of view of 16 cm.
  - The brain parenchyma and fat are suppressed well on this sequence.

Advantages: MR cisternography does not require an active CSF leak to demonstrate the site of the leak. Spontaneous leaks with or without associated cephaloceles and encephaloceles can be confidently diagnosed on MRI. The 3-D T2

DRIVE MR cisternography sequence has the advantages of effective bone and fat suppression, decreased artefacts, faster acquisition times, three-dimensional capability, and high spatial resolution, in addition to providing a very bright signal from the CSF.

Limitations: The drawback of MR cisternography is the lack of bony detail as compared to CT imaging, even though the gradient-echo images greatly improved the detail of the osseous anatomy in the skull base. But still the osseous anatomy is better appreciated with CT imaging rather than with MRI.

## NUCLEAR MEDICINE STUDIES

Radionuclide cisternography is performed with a radiotracer, the Technetium (Tc) 99 m, labelled diethylenetriamine penta-acetic acid for active CSF leaks, which has a short half-life of about 6 hours. Intermittent CSF leaks are demonstrated by a prolonged cisternography, which can be performed with a radiotracer, the Indium (In) 111, diethylenetriamine penta-acetic acid, which has a longer half-life with delayed imaging of up to 72 hrs.[5]

Indication: (i) Radionuclide cisternography is used only when CSF leak is occult; (ii) 2-transferrin cannot be collected; (iii) Cross-sectional imaging cannot locate a skull base defect.

Procedure: No matter the tracer, it is administrated via a lumbar intrathecal puncture and the patient is positioned in a Trendelenburg position, to facilitate the craniad flow of the tracer. Images are acquired when the radiotracer opacifies the basal cisterns. Images of the head and paranasal sinuses, anterior and lateral projections, are taken. The accumulation of the radiotracer within the nasal cavity or nasopharynx, suggests a CSF fistula and may detect the location of the communication.[6,7]

The extra steps to take for an undetermined CSF leak involve:

(i) The strategic endoscopic placement of nasal pledgets, 1–2 hours before intrathecal radiotracer administration, shows 76% success. It is placed in bilaterally in the spheno-ethmoidal recess, adjacent to the middle meatus, and either in the region of the cribriform plates, olfactory recess, or Eustachian tubes. About 24 hours later, the radiotracer activity within the pledgets is measured and compared to that within the serum. A CSF leak is indicated by a pledget-to-serum activity ratio of 1.5–3.0:1.[6,7]

Limitations: Very few patients are able to tolerate six intranasal pledgets for 24 hours, one or more of the cotton pledgets may fall out.

(ii) The prolonged cisternography technique shows 25% success and requires great patient compliance with the need to return for repeat imaging, sometimes up to 72 hours later, and prolonged placement of the nasal pledgets.

(iii) After administration of the radiotracer, under a controlled setting, it transiently elevates the intracranial pressure by intrathecal infusion of saline or artificial CSF. The major limitation is discomfort and headache.

Table 12.2  A diagnostic algorithm for imaging in management of CSF rhinorrhea

We do not recommend this technique in our institution, due to potential complications of headache or "opening" a defect.

(iv) Positioning the patient in a provocative position during image acquisition may improve the observation of intermittent leaks, such as prone, or in a head-hanging position.

Limitations: None of the nuclear medicine examinations can be the sole diagnostic examination, as they cannot accurately localize and characterize the defect. Therefore, such practice is reserved for complicated cases when the diagnosis is in question.

Any invasive cisternography is relatively contraindicated in patients with meningitis or elevated intracranial pressure.

We have deduced a diagnostic algorithm based on our experience (Table 12.2).

# REFERENCES

1. Lloyd KM, Del Gaudio JM, Hudgins PA. Imaging of skull base cerebrospinal fluid leaks in adults. *Radiology* 2008; 248: 725–736.
2. Glaubitt D, Haubrich J, Cordoni-Voutsas M. Detection and quantitation of intermittent CSF rhinorrhea during prolonged cisternography with 111In-DTPA. *Am J Neuroradiol* 1983; 4: 560–563.
3. Stone JA, Castillo M, Neelon B, Mukherji SK. Evaluation of CSF leaks: high-resolution CT compared with contrast-enhanced CT and radionuclide cisternography. *Am J Neuroradiol* 1999; 20: 706–712.
4. Shetty PG, Shroff MM, Sahani DV, Kirtane MV. Evaluation of high-resolution CT and MR cisternography in the diagnosis of cerebrospinal fluid fistula. *Am J Neuroradiol* 1998; 19: 633–639.

5. Vemuri NV, Karanam LS, Manchikanti V et al. Imaging review of cerebro-spinal fluid leaks. *Indian J Radiol Imag* 2017; 27(4): 441–446.
6. Shetty PG, Shroff MM, Sahani DV, Kirtane MV. Evaluation of high-resolution CT and MR cisternography in the diagnosis of cerebrospinal fluid fistula. *Am J Neuroradiol* 1998; 19(4): 633–639.
7. Mostafa BE, Khafagi A, Morcos JJ. Combined HRCT and MRI in the detection of CSF rhinorrhea. *Skull Base* 2004; 14: 157–162.

# 13

# Complications of CSF rhinorrhea

## HEMANTH VAMANSHANKAR AND JYOTIRMAY S HEGDE

Pathological leak of CSF through the nose due to a skull base bony defect and disruption of the dura and arachnoid membranes can be either traumatic or non-traumatic. This serious entity has been known to cause catastrophic consequences historically. These include meningitis, intracranial hypotension, pneumocephalus, and intracranial abscess formation.[1]

## MENINGITIS

2% of all head injury patients and 12–30% of skull base fractures develop traumatic CSF leaks. 7–30% of traumatic CSF leak cases develop meningitis, the rate of which increases as the duration of leak increases.[2] The average rate of developing meningitis in persistent CSF leak was 6.75% among various studies reviewed historically. 1–4.8% of such traumatic leaks develop severe life-threatening bacterial meningitis.[3] Recurrent bacterial meningitis is defined as multiple episodes of meningitis caused by the same organism after treatment, or two or more episodes of meningitis caused by different organisms.[4] The most common causative organisms include *Streptococcus pneumoniae* (84%), *Haemophilus influenzae* (8%), *Neisseria meningitidis* (5%), and *Staphylococcus aureus* (3%). Head trauma and recurrent meningitis are found to be more common in men.[5]

The seriousness of this dreaded complication is further highlighted given its potentially debilitating complications such as mental retardation, brain abscess, hydrocephalus, and death. Cognitive impairment, hearing loss, and focal neurological deficits can be seen as its long-term sequelae.[6,7] Incidence of death after a single episode of meningitis is as high as 21%, but this decreases with recurrent meningitis. This could possibly be due to early recognition of symptoms by the patients. Prevention of recurrent meningitis involves eliminating the risk factors of meningitis, surgical repair of defects, and vaccination against pathogens which are known to cause CNS infections.[4]

## PNEUMOCEPHALUS

Approximately 75–80% of cases of pneumocephalus are caused by trauma.[8,9] In 1884, Chiari was the first to describe this entity.[10] A reduced intracranial pressure with a defect in the dura are required for its development. The mechanism for its formation is either by negative pressure created by the leaking CSF and subsequent air entry, or a ball valve mechanism allowing air entry in a unilateral direction.[8]

Pneumocephalus usually presents with headache, hemiparesis, cranial nerve palsies, papilledema, and meningeal signs.[11] Persistent or tension pneumocephalus may present with neurological deterioration, lethargy, and headache.[12] Tension pneumocephalus is a neurosurgical emergency (most commonly seen after evacuation of a subdural hematoma), diagnosed on a CT scan as a characteristic compression of frontal lobes and widening of the interhemispheric space between the tips of the frontal lobes. This sign is called "the Mount Fuji sign" on a CT scan; it is used to differentiate tension and non-tension pneumocephalus.

Tension pneumocephalus can also occur as a result of head trauma, posterior fossa surgery in the sitting position, skull base surgery, or paranasal sinus surgery.[11,13,14]

Pneumocephalus can be managed either medically or surgically. Non-surgical method includes ventilating the patient with normobaric 100% oxygen. This causes a decrease in the volume of intracranial air and reabsorption of nitrogen into the bloodstream.[12,15] Surgical evacuation is required when features of tension pneumothorax are present, as otherwise neuronal damage occurs due to air exposure, hence further worsening brain parenchymal damage, and leading to cerebral edema.[16] Surgical evacuation is done by drilling burr holes, needle aspiration, craniotomy, or placement of a ventriculostomy and closure of the dural defect.

Patients need to be told to avoid a Valsalva maneuver or nose blowing in order to prevent recurrence.[11]

## ENCEPHALOCELE

Spontaneous CSF leaks, a variant of idiopathic intracranial hypertension (IIH), are highly prone to develop encephaloceles (in up to 50–100% of cases). They are also prone to recur following surgical repair of the defect (25–87%).[17,18] The most likely reason for this is an obstruction in the flow of CSF, which in turn causes an increase in CSF pressure in IIH patients. The hydrostatic pulsatile forces thus created act in the path of least resistance in sites of structural weakness in the skull base, such as the cribriform plate and fascia of the sellar diaphragm, thus causing thinning of the bone in these areas. Chronic thinning of the bone in these areas over many years means the patient is more prone to develop CSF leaks and encephaloceles.[19]

## DEATH

A retrospective cohort study was done by K.-H. Liao et al. comparing a study group of cohorts having traumatic brain injury with CSF leak/pneumocephaus and a control group of cohorts with traumatic brain injury without a CSF leak.[20]

The CSF leak group had more cranial nerve injuries (26.5% vs. 9.0%, p < 0.001) and intracranial hemorrhage (64.7% vs. 28.8%, p < 0.001) than cases in the comparison group. The occurrence rate of post-traumatic CSF leakage was 1.0%.[20] This was in comparison to studies done by Bell et al. who reported that 4.6% of traumatic cases developed post-traumatic CSF leakage, and Friedman et al. who reported that approximately 2% of cases treated for traumatic brain injury had post trauma CSF leakage.[21,22]

On further sub-classifying the study group into CSF otorrhea, CSF rhinorrhea, and pneumocephalus subgroups, it was found that the mortality rates were 8.5% in the otorrhea subgroup, 10.9% in the rhinorrhea subgroup, and 8.6% in the tension pneumocephalus subgroup. In the rhinorrhea subgroup, the two most common fracture sites were the frontal bone and skull base; the frontal bone was the most common fracture site in the pneumocephalus subgroup.[20]

The mortality rate of those with CSF leakage was significantly higher than for those without CSF leakage (9.0% vs. 2.8%, respectively). Among the three subgroups of post-traumatic CSF leakage, CSF rhinorrhea had a greater association with death than the other two subgroups after 1 year of follow-up.[20]

## REFERENCES

1. Elabd SS, Ahmad MM, Qetab SQ, Almalki MH. Cabergoline-induced pneumocephalus following treatment for giant invasive macroprolactinoma presenting with spontaneous cerebrospinal fluid rhinorrhea. *Clin Med Insights Endocrinol Diabetes* 2018; 11: 1179551418758640. doi: 10.1177/1179551418758640
2. Keles A, Aygencel G, Kara P et al. Posttraumatic cerebrospinal fluid leakage through forehead of a patient with a history of cranial operation: Case report. *Eur J Emerg Med* 2008; 15(3): 181–182.
3. Morgenstern Isaak A, Bach Faig A, Martínez S et al. Meningitis recurrente por defectos anat_omicos: la bacteria indica su origen. *An Pediatr* 2015; 82: 388–396.

4. Soni AJ, Modi G. Outcome of uncorrected CSF leak and consequent recurrent meningitis in a patient: A case presentation and literature review. *Br J Neurosurg.* doi: 10.1080/02688697.2018.1478063

5. Justyna J-L, Krzysztof S. Recurrent meningitis – A review of current literature. *Przegl Epidemiol* 2013; 67: 41–45.

6. Jonathon A, Friedman MD, Michael J et al. Persistent posttraumatic cerebrospinal fluid leakage. *Neurosurg Focus* 2000; 9: 1–5.

7. Van de Beek D, Schmand B, de Gans J et al. Cognitive impairment in adults with good recovery after bacterial meningitis. *J Infect Dis* 2002; 186: 1047–1052.

8. Lee J-S, Park Y-S, Kwon J-T, Suk J-S. Spontaneous pneumocephalus associated with pneumosinus dilatans. *J Korean Neurosurg Soc* 2010; 47(5): 395–398.

9. Markham JW. The clinical features of pneumocephalus based upon a survey of 284 cases with report of 11 additional cases. *Acta Neurochirurgica* 1967; 16(1–2): 1–78.

10. Chiari H. A case of acummulation of air in the ventricles of human brain. *Zeitschrift für Heilkunde* 1884; 5: 383–390.

11. Baba M, Tarar O, Syed A. A rare case of spontaneous pneumocephalus associated with nontraumatic cerebrospinal fluid leak. *Case Rep Neurol Med.* doi: 10.1155/2016/1828461

12. Paiva WS, de Andrade AF, Figueiredo EG et al. Effects of hyperbaric oxygenation therapy on symptomatic pneumocephalus. *Ther Clin Risk Manage* 2014; 10: 769–773.

13. Dabdoub CB, Salas G, Silveira Edo N, Dabdoub CF. Review of the management of pneumocephalus. *Surg Neurol Int* 2015; 6: article 155.

14. Ishiwata Y, Fujitsu K, Sekino T et al. Subdural tension pneumocephalus following surgery for chronic subdural hematoma. *J Neurosurg* 1988; 68(1): 58–61.

15. Yates H, Hamill M, Borel CO, Toung TJK. Incidence and perioperative management of tension pneumocephalus following craniofacial resection. *J Neurosurg Anesthesiol* 1994; 6 (1): 15–20.

16. Venkatesh SK, Bhargava V. Clinics in diagnostic imaging (119). Posttraumatic intracerebral pneumatocele. *Singapore Med J* 2007; 48(11): 1055–1059.

17. Badia L, Loughran S, Lund Y. Primary spontaneous cerebrospinal fluid rhinorrhea and obesity. *Am J Rhinol* 2001; 15: 117–119.

18. Casiano RR, Jassir D. Endoscopic cerebrospinal fluid rhinorrhea repair: Is a lumbar drain necessary? *Otolaryngol Head Neck Surg* 1999; 121: 745–750.

19. Schlosser RJ, Woodworth BA, Wilensky EM et al. Spontaneous cerebrospinal fluid leaks: A variant of benign intracranial hypertension. *Ann Otol Rhinol Laryngol* 2006; 115(7): 495–500.

20. Liao K, Wang J, Lin H et al. Risk of death in patients with post-traumatic cerebrospinal fluid leakage- Analysis of 1773 cases. *J Chin Med Assoc* 2016; 79(2): 58–64. doi: 10.1016/j.jcma.2015.10.002
21. Bell RB, Dierks EJ, Hormer L, Potter BE. Management of cerebrospinal fluid leak associated with craniomaxillofacial trauma. *J Oral Maxillofac Surg* 2004; 62: 676–684.
22. Friedman JA, Ebersold MJ, Quast LM. Post-traumatic cerebrospinal fluid leakage. *World J Surg* 2001; 25: 1062–1066.

# 14

# Reconstruction of skull base defects

## HEMANTH VAMANSHANKAR AND JYOTIRMAY S HEGDE

The advent of endoscopic sinonasal skull base surgeries for treating a myriad of skull base pathologies, which were previously treated by open craniotomy, and improved techniques of reconstruction with the use of grafts and flaps, have caused a drastic reduction in postoperative failures, from as high as 30–40% in the past to about 6.7–11.5%.[1,2] Reconstructions in the early 1970s were done with split thickness skin grafting, as described by Ketcham et al., which in turn caused complications like CSF leaks to the extent of 71%.[3] The pericranial flap was then described by Schafer et al. in 1986.[4] Other flaps like glabellar, temporalis, and forehead were described subsequently, but there was a need for a larger volume flap in complex resections. Myocutaneous flaps like the latissimus dorsi and pectoralis which have bulk became popular. However, what made them still unreliable was the fact that their reach to distant sites in the skull base was sometimes difficult, and the fact that necrosis at the distal part of flap was a major problem.[5] The 1980s and 1990s brought in popular microvascular techniques, which drastically reduced complication rates. The augmentation of these techniques with synthetic materials like titanium mesh and polymethylmethacrylate (PMMA), and supplements like fibrin glue, have revolutionized reconstruction techniques.[6]

Skull base defect reconstruction aims to achieve the following:

1. Provide a watertight seal so as to prevent CSF leakage from the cranial vault, hence separating the brain from the external environment.
2. Prevent ascending pharyngeal infection and a possible pneumocephalus.
3. Restore the aesthetics of forehead soft tissue and skin.
4. Repair or obliterate intracranial dead space and/or frontal sinus.
5. Provide a cover to exposed carotids.
6. Provide support for orbital contents.[5,7,8]

## CLASSIFICATION OF DEFECTS AND RECONSTRUCTIVE TECHNIQUES

Athreya el al. have classified anterior cranial fossa defects into three zones based on anatomic heterogeneity of frontal bone and differences in overlying soft tissue: firstly, low defects are those in the anterior skull base and nasal roof. Secondly, middle defects comprise the supraorbital bar, frontal sinus, and glabellar/lower forehead skin. Thirdly, high defects are those in the squamous part of the frontal bone above the frontal sinus and upper forehead/scalp soft tissues, skin (Figure 14.1).[9]

Based on the maximum diameter of defects, those which are 2.5 cm or less are termed minor defects, while those greater than 2.5 cm diameter are major defects.[10]

Defects <1 cm in size are usually repaired with avascular grafts while larger defects >3 cm are repaired by vascularized flaps.[11] The reconstruction plan, however, must be individualized to each patient. Free tissue grafts are easy to harvest with minimum donor site morbidity. However, cases involving high-flow CSF leaks, large dural defects, prior history of surgery or radiation, and benign intracranial hypertension, are more prone to graft failure and hence vascularized flaps are preferred here. Vascularized flaps are more reliable, heal faster than grafts and are for salvage purposes, when locoregional options are unavailable or have failed.[12-14] But what is more important than the size of the defect is whether the borders of the defect can be identified and exposed. This determines the ease, complexity, or impossibility of the procedure.[15]

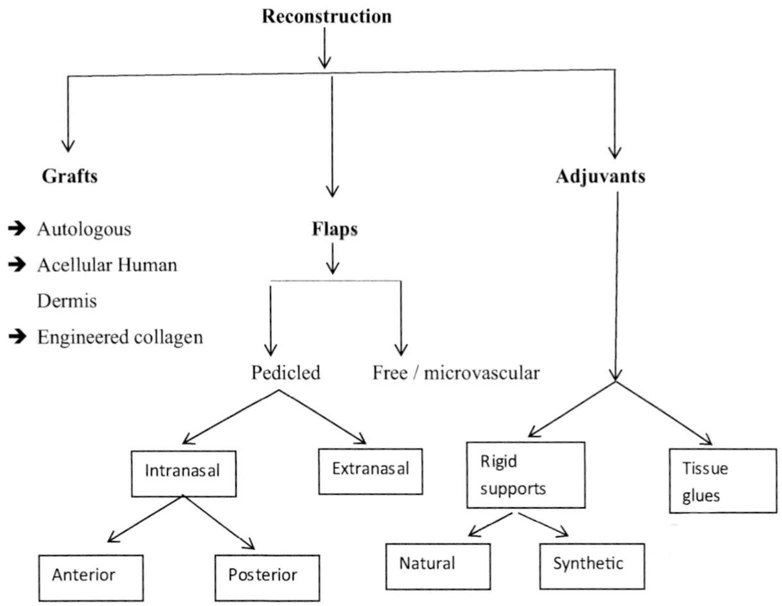

**Reconstruction**

Grafts

→ Autologous
→ Acellular Human
Dermis
→ Engineered collagen

**Flaps**

Pedicled

Free / microvascular

Intranasal

Extranasal

Anterior

Posterior

Adjuvants

Rigid supports

Tissue glues

Natural

Synthetic

Figure 14.1 Flowchart showing various modalities of reconstruction of skull base. © Jyotirmay S Hegde, Hemanth Vamanshankar.

High risk factors which may contribute to a CSF leak prior to reconstruction must be kept in mind. The presence of obesity, prior history of radiation or surgery, and Cushing's disease are considered risk factors. Anterior skull base defects are more common than clival defects. Intraoperatively high-flow CSF leaks and procedures requiring dissection into ventricles and arachnoid cisterns are associated with higher postoperative leaks.[16]

## Grafts in skull base reconstruction

For defects less than 1 cm, a variety of materials can be used as grafts. Autologous tissues like bone, cartilage, fascia, fat and free mucosal grafts have been described. These are readily available and biocompatible. They can be easily incorporated into the surrounding tissues.

Human acellular dermis grafts are popular in head and neck reconstructions, because compared to autologous tissues they do not require time for graft harvesting, and their propensity for shrinkage is low. They are relatively cheap and easy to use. Crusting, however, can be a problem with these grafts in the postoperative phase.

Collagen-based dural replacement products, termed "engineered collagen" are collagen-rich animal tissues which provide a scaffold for cell growth by promoting fibroblast ingrowth and angiogenesis.[8,17]

Autologous grafts have an overall initial success rate of 90% in leak repair and a secondary repair success rate of 97%, regardless of the type of graft chosen.[18]

Tissue glues have been extensively used in endoscopic skull base surgery, although their use has been described as "idiosyncratic and typically off label." Apart from DuraSeal that is approved by FDA as a spine sealant, none of the other tissue glue materials (e.g., Tisseal, Evicel) used are FDA-approved for endoscopic skull base surgery.[17] Eloy et al., in their case series, have described the use of vascularized septal flaps for high-flow CSF leaks with or without the use of tissue glue. They opine that the use of tissue glues may not provide an added benefit, as suggested by the fact that the only postoperative failure in the study occurred in the sealant group.[19] Complications wise, the possibility of extravasation of tissue glue into the intracranial compartment, and the inherent property of such materials to swell up after reconstitution (hence they should not be used in enclosed spaces) ought to be kept in mind.[20]

**Rigid supports** are usually indicated in cases with increased intracranial pressure, to prevent failure or recurrences.[21,22] Their use in other conditions is controversial.[23,24] The most frequently used natural materials are septal cartilage and vomer, although rib, iliac crest, split calvarial grafts, and conchal cartilage have been described. Synthetic materials include plates made of titanium mesh, or expanded polytetrafluoroethylene and bone substitutes like hydroxyapatite and polymethylmethacrylate. Synthetics have been known to have low rates of extrusion and minimal inflammatory response. Titanium mesh is malleable and safe in imaging.[25,26]

## Intranasal pedicled flaps

### POSTERIORLY BASED FLAPS

### Nasoseptal flap

Known as the workhorse of skull base reconstruction, this flap introduced in 2006 by Hadad and Bassagasteguy, is versatile for most ventral cranial base defects. It is composed of mucoperichondrium and mucoperiosteum pedicled on the nasoseptal artery branch of the posterior nasal artery, which itself is a branch of the sphenopalatine artery.[27] In the majority of cases (70%), the posterior septal artery branches into two at the sphenoid ostium level, while in 40% the branching takes place at the level of sphenopalatine foramen.[28,29] The nasoseptal flap has a wide arc of rotation and can cover defects of the anterior cranial fossa, transsphenoidal and transclival defects independently,[30] and can be harvested from either side of the nasal septum, usually the side opposite to the tumor. An endoscopic Doppler probe can be used to verify the artery's presence in the case of a wide sphenoidotomy done previously.[31]

*Technique of harvest:* After adequate vasoconstriction of septal mucosa, the superior incision is made at the sphenoid ostium, running parallel and 1 cm below the skull base, until the anterior attachment of the middle turbinate, from where it is directed upwards in the anterio-superior septum. The inferior incision is made from the superior margin of the choana, along the posterior vomer, towards the nasal floor. This is then continued anteriorly between the nasal floor and septum as far as the anterior septal margin. The two incisions are joined together and the flap is raised in a subperichondrial and subperiosteal plane, preserving the vascular pedicle. Dissection may be difficult in the presence of a deviated septum or spur. The pedicle should be protected from excessive cautery and microdebrider use. Mucosa of the floor of the nasal cavity can also be included in the flap if a wider flap is desired[32] (Figure 14.2 A). Thorp et al., in their series of 151 repairs using the nasoseptal flap in various pathologies, have reported a postoperative leak rate of 3.3%, no reports of flap death, and no recurrent leak after 3 months.[33] Crusting and synechae formation at the donor site is a postoperative problem,

## FLAPS FOR SKULL BASE RECONSTRUCTION

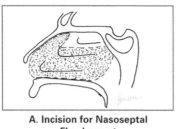

A. Incision for Nasoseptal
Flap harvest

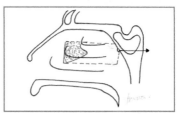

B. Posterior Nasoseptal Flap

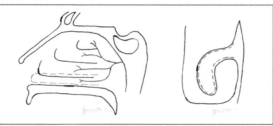

C. Sagittal & Coronal Images showing Incision for inferior turbinate flap

D. PERICRANIAL FLAP

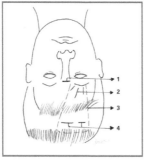

1. 1 cm Glabellar Incision
2. Marking Of Arterial Pedicles
3. Outline Of Proposed Pericranial Flap
4. 2 cm & 1 cm Scalp Incisions

Figure 14.2 (A) Nasoseptal flap. (B) Posterior nasoseptal flap. (C) Inferior turbinate flap. (D) Pericranial flap. © Jyotirmay S Hegde, Hemanth Vamanshankar.

which can be minimized with the use of mucosal grafts over exposed cartilage or silastic splints kept for 2–3 weeks. An advantage of the nasoseptal flap is its use as a "rescue flap" and the fact that it can be reused in concurrent surgery.[32]

## Inferior turbinate flap

This is based on the inferior turbinate artery, a branch of the posterior lateral nasal artery-branch of sphenopalatine artery, first described by Fortes in 2007.[34] The flap is harvested by first identifying the sphenopalatine artery at its foramen, and then following the posterior lataeral nasal into the inferior turbinate. The artery usually enters the postero-superior aspect of the inferior turbinate in a descending fashion, 1–1.5 cm from the posterior tip. The upper incision is made just above the inferior turbinate, and the lower is done at its inferior margin. The two incisions are joined by a vertical incision at the head of inferior turbinate, and the mucoperichondrium is lifted off the turbinate bone. The inferior incision can be made into the inferior meatus if more area is required (Figure 14.2 C). Crusting is usually present for 3–4 weeks. This flap is usually suited for clival and sellar defects.[35] This flap, however, has a decreased length and surface area as compared to other locoregional flaps.[36,37]

## Middle turbinate flap

This flap is based on the sphenopalatine and anterior septal artery branches. Adequate coverage is provided by this flap for transtubercular, transplanar, and/ or transsellar defects.[38] For harvesting the flap, a vertical incision is made on the anterior aspect of the middle turbinate, starting from just below the cribriform plate level, after adequate infiltration. The mucosa is carefully elevated without destabilizing the turbinate, as far as the posterior pedicle. After removal of the bone, a horizontal incision is made at the axilla of the turbinate and the flap is mobilized.[38,39] Postoperatively, periodic removal of clots and crusting may be necessary until the mucosa heals. The presence of bullous turbinates, highly variable pneumatization, and the small surface area of coverage are the challenges in using this flap.[39]

## Posterior nasoseptal flap

Barger et al. have described a modification of the nasoseptal flap, with the advantage of being much smaller than the latter, composed mainly of mucosal tissue that is otherwise discarded during posterior septectomy (hence the flap is routinely raised in all cases whether required or not), and having lesser crusting postoperatively. The technique involves the lateralization of all three turbinates after nasal decongestion. A vertical incision of the mid-nasal septum corresponding to the anterior aspect of middle turbinate is made. Two horizontal posterior incisions are then made from the limbs of the vertical: the superior one just below the cribriform plate, and the inferior one along the maxillary crest. The mucoperiosteum is then raised posteriorly until the sphenoid ostium (Figure 14.2 B). A similar flap may be raised on the other nostril also if required. The authors have reported a 97.7% success rate of CSF leak closure using this technique.[40]

## ANTERIORLY BASED FLAPS

Limitations of the posterior-based flap length, due to which adequate coverage was not being provided to extremely anterior sites like the posterior frontal table and anterior cribriform, and tethering of the flap pedicle by sphenopalatine foramen have highlighted the need for further research, which have in turn paved the way for the development of anteriorly based flaps.

### Bipedicled anterior septal flap

The anterior nose is composed of many small caliber vessels, two of which (the nasopalatine artery and septal branch of the superior labial artery) when put together form the bipedicled anterior septal flap. Radioanatomic measurement studies on cadavers by Bleier et al. have found this flap feasible for the reconstruction of anterior skull base defects, frontal beak, and the posteror frontal table. The flap, however, needs to be harvested prior to the surgery and stored in the floor of the nose. It is mainly used in cases where a prior FESS with a wide sphenoidotomy was done, and the status of the posterior septal artery may not be known.[41]

### Anterior lateral nasal wall flaps

The anterior inferior turbinate artery flap based on the anterior ethmoid artery was described in 2012 by Gil and Margalir. This anterior-based mucoperichondrial flap can incorporate the entire length of the inferior turbinate and can cover defects in the ethmoid roof, cribriform plate, and the posterior table of the frontal sinus.[42]

## Extranasal pedicled flaps

### PERICRANIAL FLAP

The most common second-line vascular flap used after the nasoseptal flap, based on the supraorbital and supratrochlear arteries. Used extensively for reconstruction during the external approaches for skull base lesions, its role has again been keenly studied in the endoscopic era, as by making a small nasionectomy incision, it can be incorporated easily into anterior skull base defects. The flap offers a large surface area and length for anterior skull base defects; its harvesting is less technically demanding, is cosmetically favourable, and offers better radioresistance than most other pedicled flaps. Harvesting of this flap is nonetheless difficult in persons with a protruding forehead, low hairline, and short forehead.[8]

Zanation et al. have described a minimally invasive endoscopic technique for pericranial flap harvesting. A 2 cm midline and 1 cm lateral port incision are made in the hairline. A Doppler ultrasound is used to identify the supratrochlear and supraorbital arteries and the pedicle is marked. A needle-tip cautery bent to 90 degrees at the tip is used to incise the pericranium under endoscopic guidance; the periosteal dissector is used to raise the flap from the skull posteriorly to anteriorly. A horizontal glabellar incision is made and dissected as far as the periosteum (Figure 14.2 D). Diamond burrs are used to create a defect of 4 mm x 1.5 cm, through which the pericranial flap is transposed. A suction drain is kept to prevent scalp hematoma. Bone removal at the nasion is ideal for this procedure as it corresponds to the skull base and is not palpable or seen. Complications are minimal with this procedure: scalp edema and pain are reported.[43]

### TEMPOROPARIETAL FASCIAL FLAP

This fan-shaped flap based on the superficial temporal artery is suitable for defects involving the sella, parasella, and clivus. Its use in anterior skull base defects is limited as it must rotate 90 degrees and pass through the pterygopalatine fossa. Patients who have undergone skull base and sinonasal radiotherapy particularly benefit from the use of this flap as it does not come into the irradiated field. However, the need for an additional external incision and the risk of developing alopecia at the site, and the possibility of injuring the facial nerve, must be kept in mind while harvesting this flap.[11,44,45]

### PALATAL FLAP

Based on the greater palatine artery, this mucoperiosteal flap is harvested from the hard palate, and tunnelled through the greater palatine foramen into the nasal cavity. The possibility of an oroantral fistula formation as a complication should be taken into consideration.[46,47]

### PEDICLED FACIAL BUCCINATORS FLAP

Described by Rivera-Serrano et al., it can be used either as an entirely muscular flap or like a myomucosal flap. Pedicled on the facial artery, it is said to cover defects of the planum sphenoidale and anterior skull base. It can be harvested as a myomucosal flap or just muscular flap. Potential complications of this flap include facial/dental paraesthesia, the possibility of oral contamination in the surgical field, and persistent epiphora.[48]

### OCCIPITAL GALEOPERICRANIAL FLAP

Based on the occipital artery and used mainly for posterior skull base defects.[49] Pedicle dissection begins from the overlying neck and usually has a consistent anatomic location. Initial requirements for flap placement are a wide endoscopic maxillary antrostomy, posterior maxillary wall removal, and inferior aspect of pterygoid plate removal. The flap is tunnelled along the inferomedial aspect of the medial pterygoid muscle.[50]

## Microvascular free flaps

### RADIAL FOREARM FLAP

This is an extremely versatile flap based on the radial artery and its vena comitantes. Location of the pedicle is very consistent and is identified between the brachioradialis and flexor carpi radialis muscles. A preoperative Allen's test must be done prior to harvesting this flap to prevent the possibility of hand ischemia postoperatively. Large defects in the skull base may not benefit from this flap due to its limited surface area.[51]

### RECTUS ABDOMINIS MYOCUTANEOUS FLAP

Based on the inferior epigastric artery and vein, it is harvested through a paramedian abdominal incision. A pedicle of 12–15 cm can be obtained from this flap. Muscle lining in the anterior cranial fossa can be augmented with the use of an anterior rectus sheath or fascia lata graft. The epigastric vessels are anastomosed to facial vessels through a subcutaneous tunnel in the cheek or to superficial temporal vessels through a burr hole in the lateral wall of the frontal bone. The muscle has the benefit of filling into irregular cavities of the skull base and the bulk prevents CSF leaks. A rich blood supply also helps in the diffusion of antibiotics into the reconstruction area, with rapid uneventful healing.[52]

### LATISSIMUS DORSI FLAP

Based on the thoracodorsal vessels, this flat muscle provides for a large quality of well vascularised tissue, using virtually the entire musculature. However, since the harvest has to be done in the lateral decubitus position, it cannot be performed at the same time as the primary procedure, hence increasing operative time. The muscle also atrophies over a period of time, and so may not be able to fill in dead space. Serratus anterior muscle, if included in such a flap, may cause winging of the scapula.[51]

### ANTEROLATERAL THIGH FLAP

Based on the perforators of the descending branch of the lateral circumflex femoral artery. A vertical line from the anterior superior iliac spine to the superolateral border of the patella is used to represent intermuscular septum between the vastus lateralis and rectus femoris. Doppler is used to identify cutaneous vessels over the midpoint of the line. Flap dissection starts from the medial aspect, incising over the rectus femoris, through the deep fascia, until the intermuscular septum. The lateral circumflex femoral is found here. The lateral incision is done and a 2 cm cuff of vastus lateralis muscle is taken with the flap, once the pedicle is stabilized. The flap has a long vascular pedicle and the donor site has minimum morbidity.[51]

## CLOSURE OF DEFECTS

A multilayer approach for the closure of skull base defects is ideal in reconstruction. An initial underlay graft using fascia, cartilage, collagen dural substitute, or acellular dermal allograft are suitable. Mucosal grafts are then placed in an overlay fashion. The latter are avoided being placed intracranially due to reports of mucocele formation.[53] These are further bolstered intranasally using tissue glue and an expandable sponge packing or the use of a Foley catheter balloon. Abdominal fat can be used to obliterate dead space and as an additional bolster.[16]

A recent study exploring the factors affecting outcomes of reconstruction of anterior skull base defects showed that factors like the sex of the patient, pathology treated, previous skull base surgery, the presence of multiple defects, size of defect, reconstruction technique employed, material used for reconstruction, and exposure to radiotherapy did not show any statistical significance. What was statistically significant was the year in which surgery was performed, which meant there was a clear reduction in the failure cases over the years.[15]

Skull base reconstruction requires a multidisciplinary approach, with otolaryngology, neurosurgical, maxillofacial, and plastic surgical teams working in tandem. Navigation systems, surgical refinements, and advanced endoscopic techniques have clearly contributed to bring about a drastic reduction in failures and improving the quality of life of such patients. Reconstruction forms an integral form of treatment post-removal of the skull base pathology, and equal importance has to be given to reconstruction with regards to the primary surgery. Another feature which is unique to skull base reconstruction is the fact that the flaps here are harvested prior to the actual surgery, again emphasizing the importance of the reconstruction procedure.

## TAKE-HOME POINTS

- Reconstructions using local or microvascular flaps in skull base have caused a huge positive impact to the post-operative status and quality of life in these patients.
- Reconstruction options are many: various types of grafts and pedicled, or microvascular flaps with adjuvants like tissue glues are available.
- The nasoseptal and pericranial flaps are the first and second choice flaps in most cases.
- A multi-layered closure is now considered the treatment of choice in all skull base defects for providing optimum results.
- Reconstruction in skull base is done prior to the surgical procedure intended.

## REFERENCES

1. Soudry E, Turner JH, Nayak JV, Hwang PH. Endoscopic reconstruction of surgically created skull base defects: A systematic review. *Otolaryngol Head Neck Surg* 2014; 150(5):730–8.
2. Harvey RJ, Parmar P, Sacks R, Zanation AM. Endoscopic skull base reconstruction of large dural defects: A systematic review of published evidence. *Laryngoscope* 2012; 122(2):452–9.
3. Ketcham AS, Wilkins RH, Van Buren JM, Smith RR. A combined intra-cranial facial approach to the paranasal sinuses. *Am J Surg* 1963; 106:698–703.
4. Schaefer SD, Close LG, Mickey BE. Axial subcutaneous scalp flaps in the reconstruction of the anterior cranial fossa. *Arch Otolaryngol Head Neck Surg* 1986; 112:745–9.

5. Trivedi NP, Kuriakose MA, Iyer S. Reconstruction in skull base surgery: Review of current concepts. *Indian J Plast Surg* 2007; 40:S52–9.
6. Reinard K, Basheer A, Jones L et al. Surgical technique for repair of complex anterior skull base defects. *Surg Neurol Int* 2015; 6:20.
7. Vargo JD, Przylecki W, Camarata PJ, Andrews BT. Classification and microvascular flap selection for anterior cranial fossa reconstruction. *J Reconstr Microsurg* 2018; 34:590–600. doi: 10.1055/s-0038-1649520
8. Rawal RB, Ambrose EC, Patel MR, Zanation AM. Advances in reconstruction of the skull base. *Curr Otorhinolaryngol Rep* 2013; 1:191–6.
9. Athreya S. The frontal bone in the genus Homo: A survey of functional and phylogenetic sources of variation. *J Anthropol Sci* 2012; 90:59–80.
10. Hoffmann TK, El Hindy N, Müller OM et al. Vascularised local and free flaps in anterior skull base reconstruction. *Eur Arch Otorhinolaryngol* 2013; 270:899–907.
11. Zanation AM, Thorp BD, Parmar P et al. Reconstructive options for endoscopic skull base surgery. *Otolaryngol Clin North Am* 2011; 44(5):1201–22.
12. Snyderman CH, Kassam AB, Carrau R et al. Endoscopic reconstruction of cranial base defects following endonasal skull base surgery. *Skull Base* 2007; 17:73–8.
13. Hegazy HM, Carrau RL, Snyderman CH et al. Transnasal endoscopic repair of cerebrospinal fluid rhinorrhea: A meta-analysis. *Laryngoscope* 2000; 110:1166–72.
14. Woodworth BA, Prince A, Chiu AG et al. Spontaneous CSF leaks: A paradigm for definitive repair and management of intracranial hypertension. *Otolaryngol Head Neck Surg* 2008; 138:715–20.
15. Turri-Zanoni M, Zocchi J, Lambertoni A et al. Endoscopic endonasal reconstruction of anterior skull base defects: What factors really affect the outcomes? *World Neurosurg* 2018; 116:e436–43. doi: 10.1016/j.wneu.2018.04.225
16. Kim GG, Hang AX, Mitchell CA, Zanation AM. Pedicled extranasal flaps in skull base reconstruction. In Bleier BS (Ed.), *Comprehensive Techniques in CSF Leak Repair and Skull Base Reconstruction*. Basel, Switzerland: Karger Publishers. 2013; Vol. 74, pp. 71–80.
17. Prickett KK, Wise SK. Grafting materials in skull base reconstruction. In Bleier BS (Ed.), *Comprehensive Techniques in CSF Leak Repair and Skull Base Reconstruction*. Basel, Switzerland: Karger Publishers. 2013; Vol. 74, pp. 24–32.
18. Rawal RB, Kimple AJ, Dugar DR et al. Minimizing morbidity in endoscopic pituitary surgery: Outcomes of the novel nasoseptal rescue flap technique. *Otolaryngol Head Neck Surg* 2012; 147(3):434–7.
19. Eloy JA, Choudhry OJ, Friedel ME, Kuperan AB, Liu JK. Endoscopic nasoseptal flap repair of skull base defects: Is addition of a dural sealant necessary? *Otolaryngol Head Neck Surg* 2012; 147:161–6.

20. Epstein NE. Dural repair with four spinal sealants: Focused review of the manufacturers' inserts and the current literature. *Spine J* 2010; 10:1065–8.
21. Wang EW, Vandergrift WA 3rd, Schlosser RJ. Spontaneous CSF leaks. *Otolaryngol Clin North Am* 2011; 44:845–56.
22. Wise SK, Schlosser RJ. Evaluation of spontaneous nasal cerebrospinal fluid leaks. *Curr Opin Otolaryngol Head Neck Surg* 2007; 15:28–34.
23. Esposito F, Dusick JR, Fatemi N, Kelly DF. Graded repair of cranial base defects and cerebrospinal fluid leaks in transsphenoidal surgery. *Neurosurgery* 2007; 60 Supplement 2:295–303.
24. Harvey RJ, Nogueira JF, Schlosser RJ et al. Closure of large skull base defects after endoscopic transnasal craniotomy. *J Neurosurg* 2009; 111:371–79.
25. Costantino PD, Hiltzik DH, Sen C et al. Sphenoethmoid cerebrospinal fluid leak repair with hydroxyapatite cement. *Arch Otolaryngol Head Neck Surg* 2001; 127:588–93.
26. Moliterno JA, Mubita LL, Huang C, Boockvar JA. High-viscosity poly-methylmethacrylate cement for endoscopic anterior cranial base reconstruction. *J Neurosurg* 2010; 113:1100–105.
27. Hadad G, Bassagasteguy L, Carrau RL et al. A novel reconstructive technique after endoscopic expanded endonasal approaches: Vascular pedicle nasoseptal flap. *Laryngoscope* 2006; 116(10):1882–6.
28. Babin E, Moreau S, de Rugy MG et al. Anatomic variations of the arteries of the nasal fossa. *Otolaryngol Head Neck Surg* 2003; 128:236–39.
29. Pinheiro-Neto CD, Ramos HF, Peris-Celda M et al. Study of the naso-septal flap for endoscopic anterior cranial base reconstruction. *Laryngoscope* 2011; 121:2514–20.
30. Pinheiro-Neto CD, Prevedello DM, Carrau RL et al. Improving the design of the pedicled nasoseptal flap for skull base reconstruction: A radioana-tomic study. *Laryngoscope* 2007; 117(9):1560–9.
31. Pinheiro-Neto CD, Carrau RL, Prevedello DM et al. Use of acoustic Doppler sonography to ascertain the feasibility of the pedicled naso-septal flap after prior bilateral sphenoidotomy. *Laryngoscope* 2010; 120:1798–801.
32. Pinheiro-Neto CD, Snyderman CH. Nasoseptal flap. In Bleier BS (Ed.), *Comprehensive Techniques in CSF Leak Repair and Skull Base Reconstruction.* Basel, Switzerland: Karger Publishers, 2013. Vol. 74, pp. 42–55.
33. Thorp B, Sreenath S, Ebert C, Zanation A. Endoscopic skull base recon-struction: A review and clinical case series of 152 vascularized flaps used for surgical skull base defects in the setting of intraoperative cerebrospi-nal fluid leak. *Neurosurgery* 2014; 37:E4.
34. Fortes FS, Carrau RL, Snyderman CH et al. The posterior pedicle infe-rior turbinate flap: A new vascularized flap for skull base reconstruction. *Laryngoscope* 2007; 117:1329–32.

35. Suh JD, Chiu AG. Sphenopalatine-derived pedicled flaps. In Bleier BS (Ed.), *Comprehensive Techniques in CSF Leak Repair and Skull Base Reconstruction.* Basel, Switzerland: Karger Publishers. 2013. Vol. 74, pp. 56–63.

36. Yip J, Macdonald KI, Lee J et al. The inferior turbinate flap in skull base reconstruction. *J Otolaryngol Head Neck Surg* 2013; 42(1):6.

37. Harvey RJ, Sheahan PO, Schlosser RJ. Inferior turbinate pedicle flap for endoscopic skull base defect repair. *Am J Rhinol Allergy* 2009; 23(5):522–6.

38. Prevedello DM, Barges-Coll J, Fernandez-Miranda JC et al. Middle turbinate flap for skull base reconstruction: Cadaveric feasibility study. *Laryngoscope* 2009; 119(11):2094–8.

39. Simal Julián JA, Miranda Lloret P, Cárdenas Ruiz-Valdepeñas E et al. Middle turbinate vascularized flap for skull base reconstruction after an expanded endonasal approach. *Acta Neurochir* 2011; 153:1827–32.

40. Barger J, Siow M, Kader M et al. The posterior nasoseptal flap: A novel technique for closure after endoscopic transsphenoidal resection of pituitary adenomas. *Surg Neurol Int* 2018; 9:32.

41. Meier JC, Bleier BS. Anteriorly based pedicled flaps for skull base reconstruction. In Bleier BS (Ed.), *Comprehensive Techniques in CSF Leak Repair and Skull Base Reconstruction.* Basel, Switzerland: Karger Publishers. 2013. Vol. 74, pp. 64–70.

42. Gil Z, Margalir N. Anteriorly based inferior turbinate flap for endoscopic skull base reconstruction. *Otolaryngol Head Neck Surg* 2012; 146:842–47.

43. Zanation AM, Snyderman CH, Carrau RL et al. Minimally invasive endoscopic pericranial flap: A new method for endonasal skull base reconstruction. *Laryngoscope* 2009; 119:13–8.

44. Harvey RJ, Parmar P, Sacks R, Zanation AM. Endoscopic skull base reconstruction of large dural defects: A systematic review of published evidence. *Laryngoscope* 2012; 122:452–9.

45. Patel MR, Stadler ME, Snyderman CH et al. How to choose? Endoscopic skull base reconstructive options and limitations. *Skull Base* 2010; 20:397–404.

46. Oliver CL, Hackman TG, Carrau RL et al. Palatal flap modifications allow pedicled reconstruction of the skull base. *Laryngoscope* 2008; 118(12):2102–6.

47. Hackman T, Chicoine MR, Uppaluri R. Novel application of the palatal island flap for endoscopic skull base reconstruction. *Laryngoscope* 2009; 119(8):1463–6.

48. Rivera-Serrano CM, Oliver CL, Sok J et al. Pedicled facial buccinator (FAB) flap: A new flap for reconstruction of skull base defects. *Laryngoscope* 2010; 120:1922–30.

49. Rivera-Serrano CM, Snyderman CH, Carrau RL et al. Transparapharyngeal and transpterygoid transposition of a pedicled occipital galeopericranial flap: A new flap for skull base reconstruction. *Laryngoscope* 2011; 121:914–22.
50. Dogliotti PL, Bennun RD. Occipitoparietal bone flap for mandibular reconstruction. *J Craniofac Surg* 1995; 6:249–54.
51. Herr MW, Lin DT. Microvascular free flaps in skull base reconstruction. In Bleier BS (Ed.), *Comprehensive Techniques in CSF Leak Repair and Skull Base Reconstruction*. Basel, Switzerland: Karger Publishers. 2013; Vol. 74, pp. 81–91.
52. Yamada A, Harii K, Ueda K, Asato H. Free rectus abdominis muscle reconstruction of the anterior skull base. *Br J Plastic Surg* 1992; 45:302–6.
53. Ting JY. Metson R. Free graft techniques in skull base reconstruction. In Bleier BS (Ed.), *Comprehensive Techniques in CSF Leak Repair and Skull Base Reconstruction*. Basel, Switzerland: Karger Publishers, 2013. Vol. 74, pp. 33–41.

# 15

# Recent advances in the management of CSF rhinorrhea

## HEMANTH VAMANSHANKAR AND JYOTIRMAY S HEGDE

## TAU PROTEINS AS A MARKER IN CSF RHINORRHEA

Tau proteins are a group of highly soluble intraneural protein isoforms that play a primary role in maintaining the stability of microtubules in axons. They were first identified in 1975, and their increased concentration in CSF is a diagnostic biomarker for Alzheimer's disease.[1] Their concentration in serum is much lower, with a CSF:serum ratio of 10:1, hence they are almost undetectable in other body fluids.[2] Oudart et al. assessed 26 patients with a history of CSF rhinorrhea. Tau protein concentration in the collected samples were assessed by a sandwich ELISA, and were found to have a mean value of 711 ng/L in the CSF rhinorrhea group, as compared to a mean value of 87 ng/L in the non-CSF leakage group (viral or allergic rhinitis). The main advantage of tau protein markers is in the fact that their value is not affected by blood contamination, as compared to other markers like $\beta2$-transferrin and $\beta$-trace protein. This may be of advantage in cases of CSF rhinorrhea that occur following head trauma.[3]

## ROLE OF LEUKOCYTE – PLATELET RICH FIBRIN IN RECONSTRUCTION OF CSF RHINORRHEA DEFECTS

Choukroun et al. in 2001 developed the first protocols of leukocyte and platelet-rich fibrin.[4] Platelet-rich concentrates are divided into two subgroups: platelet rich-plasma and platelet-rich fibrin, both being available in their leukocyte-enriched or pure form. These are known to release a variety of growth factors, cytokines including a platelet-derived growth factor and tumor growth factor β, a vascular endothelial growth factor, and an insulin-like growth factor.[4] All these factors in turn help in the surgical site healing.[5,6]

A patient's autologous blood is taken and centrifuged. This induces the formation of coagulation cascade and platelet activation. Fibrinogen is converted to fibrin by the action of thrombin. The resultant fibrin clot gets separated from the red blood cell layer formed at the bottom of the tube. These are then compressed and used in multilayer reconstruction grafts. They are easy to prepare, inexpensive, easy to insert and manipulate, and act like a solid autograft ensuring an immediate watertight seal unlike fibrin glue. Also, no anaphylactic reaction is noted as it is used from the patient's own blood.[5,6]

## RECONSTRUCTION OF SKULL BASE DEFECTS

A major challenge during skull base reconstruction is the spatial conformation of the skull base defect, especially when the defect extends over different compartments of the base of the skull. Effective strategies of reconstruction like gasket seal and its modifications would be ineffective in such defects, due to uneven edges. Essayed et al. have conceptualized a 3-D printing and intraoperative neuronavigation technique for the tailoring of such defects. Although this technique was undertaken in three human cadavers, it offers promising future outcomes. Pre- and post-op (after endoscopic endonasal creation of a defect in the skull base), thin cut volumetric bone window CT scans were done. Two models were then conceptualized: one based on a pre-operative CT scan (ex-model), and the other, a tailored model (T-model). A 3-D model was reconstructed based on the defect, having a rigid core, flexible edges, and an incorporated graded material interface between the rigid and flexible phases. After modeling, handles were added to the inferior nasal surface which helped as a landmark for navigation, and for maneuvring the model into the defect. The T-models were directly implanted into the bony defects, while the ex-models were tailored using a navigation technique. The results showed that although T-models were not able to provide a stable reconstruction, the ex-models gave a stable and successful closure of defects in all three cadavers using a navigation transfer. The two issues in this technique were the intraoperative time consumed for the procedure, and the issue of sterility during the procedure.[7]

3-D printing and navigation have offered a realistic option for overcoming challenges in multi-layered reconstruction, considering the anatomical locations of the defect, important neurovascular structures surrounding it, and the specific nasal and bony anatomy of each patient.

# ADVANCES IN NEURONAVIGATION AND NEURORADIOLOGY

The future may offer the possibility of combining i-CR and i-MR imaging techniques to give better image quality intraoperatively, with less intraoperative radiation burden. Imaging of histological specimens in 3-D without the need for staining or sectioning may be a future possibility with the advent of ultrasonographic scanning at high frequencies, namely microscanning. The combination of PET and SPECT in the operating room itself would also offer excellent intraoperative imaging guidance to the surgical procedure.[8,9]

# ASSESSING THE VIABILITY OF HADAD FLAP POST-OPERATIVELY

The skull base defect reconstruction is very important to prevent post-operative complications. The vascular pedicled-nasoseptal flap (Hadad-Bassagasteguy flap) is commonly used in reconstruction of the defect. A post-operative contrast-enhanced MRI examination is a very useful tool to assess the viability of the vascularised flap. An axial, sagittal, and coronal T1 and T2, pre- and post-contrast fat saturation T1 images are examined. A uniformly detectable flap covering over the skull base defects form an "open cup" appearance, which is isointense on T1-weighted/fat-suppressed images to the adjacent nasal mucosa and hyperintense on T2-weighted images, being suggestive of a viable Hadad flap.[10]

# REFERENCES

1. Oudart J, Zucchini L, Maquart F et al. Tau protein as a possible marker of cerebrospinal fluid leakage in cerebrospinal fluid rhinorrhoea: A pilot study. *Biochem Med* 2017;27(3):030703. doi: 10.11613/BM.2017.030703

2. Zetterberg H. Tau in biofluids - Relation to pathology, imaging and clinical features. *Neuropathol Appl Neurobiol* 2017;43:194–9. doi: 10.1111/nan.12378

3. Reiber H. Dynamics of brain-derived proteins in cerebrospinal fluid. *Clin Chim Acta* 2001;310:173–86. doi: 10.1016/S0009-8981(01)00573-3

4. Zhao Q, Ding Y, Si T. Platelet-rich fibrin in plastic surgery. *OA Evid Based* 2013;1:3.

5. Soldatova L, Campbell RG, Elkhatib AH et al. Role of leukocyte–platelet-rich fibrin inendoscopic endonasal skull base surgery defect reconstruction. *J Neurol Surg B* 2017;78:059–62. doi: 10.1055/s-0036-1584894

6. Khafagy YW, Elfattah AM, Moneir W, Salem EH. Leukocyte- and platelet-rich fibrin: A new graft material in endoscopic repair of spontaneous CSF leaks. *Eur Arch of Oto-Rhino-Laryngol* 2018;257:2245–52. doi: 10.1007/s00405-018-5048-7

7. Essayed WI, Unadkat P, Hosny A et al. 3D printing and intraoperative neuronavigation tailoring for skull base reconstruction after extended endoscopic endonasal surgery: Proof of concept. *J Neurosurg* 2018;130(1):248–55.

8. Enchev Y. Neuronavigation: Geneology, reality, and prospects. *Neurosurg Focus* 2009;27(3):E11.

9. Wells PN. Advances in ultrasound: From microscanning to telerobotics. *Br J Radiol* 2000;73:1138–47.

10. Jyotirmay H, Saxena SK, Ramesh AS, Nagarajan K, Bhat S. Assessing the viability of Hadad flap by postoperative contrast-enhanced magnetic resonance imaging. *J Clin Diagn Res* 2017;11(6):MC01–3.

# Index

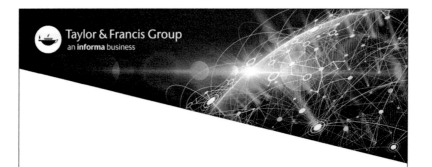

# Taylor & Francis eBooks

## www.taylorfrancis.com

A single destination for eBooks from Taylor & Francis
with increased functionality and an improved user
experience to meet the needs of our customers.

90,000+ eBooks of award-winning academic content in
Humanities, Social Science, Science, Technology, Engineering,
and Medical written by a global network of editors and authors.

## TAYLOR & FRANCIS EBOOKS OFFERS:

A streamlined
experience for
our library
customers

A single point
of discovery
for all of our
eBook content

Improved
search and
discovery of
content at both
book and
chapter level

## REQUEST A FREE TRIAL
### support@taylorfrancis.com

 Routledge
Taylor & Francis Group

 CRC Press
Taylor & Francis Group